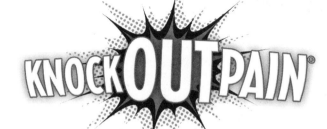

Secrets to Maintain a Healthy Back

Wishing You a Healthy and Happy new year
P. Bragg

WINIFRED BRAGG, MD

This book is written based upon my twenty years of clinical experience of treating thousands of people with back problems. The goal of this book is to educate people about low back pain and to offer strategies for pain relief.

This book cannot offer any guarantee about the resolution of your back problem or your pain. All case histories presented as examples herein are offered for teaching purposes only. In each instance, facts were changed to protect privacy. This book is not a substitution for an evaluation by your physician. An examination by a health care professional is always appropriate for the evaluation of your back pain. The recommendations in this book may differ from those of your health care provider, and they are not meant to replace any diagnosis or medical treatment by your provider.

This book is dedicated to my mom for her support and continuous encouragement that kept me on track while writing this book. It is also dedicated to my patients who have given me the honor of being their physician.

Table of Contents

Introduction

Over the past 20 years, I have treated thousands of people with back pain. I have noticed that back pain comes at inopportune times. It destroys vacations, work, traveling, outings, holidays, and special occasions. By age 55, approximately 80% of us will have had back pain at some point in our lives.

This guide was created to address those needs. It is illustrative and demonstrates the appropriate way to perform many activities of daily living, which if performed incorrectly, can result in low back pain. By following these recommendations, you can increase the likelihood of maintaining a healthy back. The best cure for back pain is to prevent it. You will learn about the basics of the spine (back), and more importantly, how to prevent back pain. But prevention is up to you.

What contributes to back pain? Simply remember what I call the O's Of LIFE ®:

O's of Life®

Primary Factors that Contribute to Back Pain

- Older age
- Osteoarthritis
- Osteoporosis
- Obesity/Overweight
- Overuse
- Occupational risks

Remember, poor conditioning and improper use of the back can contribute to back pain.

This book answers some of the following questions:

- When is surgery necessary? You will understand that surgery does not get rid of your pain forever.
- What should you do when you are away from home on vacation if back pain should suddenly strike you?
- What can I do to prevent back pain?
- How does physical therapy help with back pain?
- Can an epidural injection relieve my back pain?
- When should I seek medical attention for back pain?
- Does pain management mean I will be treated with narcotics?

Keep reading; the answers to these questions and more are in this book. Don't you dare leave home without it. I want people to carry this book with them at all times to help them prevent back pain. I also encourage you to read this book before you go to the doctor to enhance your communication with your physician.

SECTION I

Learn the Basics of the Lumbar Spine

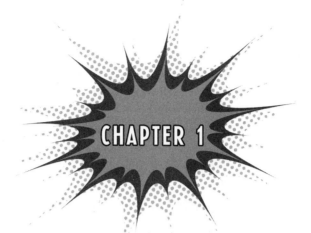

What You Need to Know About the Basics of Back Pain

WHO GETS LOW BACK PAIN?

Low back pain is widespread and is one of the most frequent reasons people seek health care. It is estimated that 80%—four out of five of us—will experience back pain by age 55, and it is the leading cause of long-term work disability.

While it is often thought that low back pain is primarily a condition of blue-collar workers, it is actually "collar blind," affecting both blue- and white-collar workers alike. And it affects both men and women. However, it is reported that women have more back pain than men.

WHAT ARE THE SYMPTOMS OF BACK PAIN?

Back pain can feel like a dull, constant ache or can manifest as a sharp pain that makes it hard to move. Symptoms of back pain may range from a muscle ache to shooting or stabbing pain, limited flexibility and range of motion, or an inability to stand straight. Back pain can either be acute or chronic in nature. Acute back pain comes on suddenly and can last from a few days to a few weeks.

WHAT ARE THE CAUSES OF LOW BACK PAIN?

Most acute back pain is the result of trauma to the lower back or a disorder such as arthritis. Pain from trauma may be caused by a sports injury, work around the house or in the garden, or a sudden jolt such as a car accident or other stress on spinal bones and tissues.

Back pain can also occur from simple things or any activity that requires long periods of sitting, lifting, bending, twisting, or repetitive motions; all increase the risk of having back pain.

Some might ask, why is low back pain so common?

The spine is composed of bones, muscles, ligaments, tendons, and discs. Back pain arises if a problem occurs with any of these structures.

There are many causes of low back pain, as you will read about in section II.

SECTION II

Ten Common Causes
of Low Back Pain

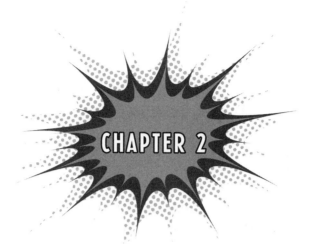

CHAPTER 2

Mom Knows Best: Get Rid of Bad Posture and Poor Body Mechanics

HOW DOES YOUR POSTURE AFFECT BACK PAIN?

Using bad posture and poor body mechanics while performing the activities of daily living can cause back pain. Lifting a heavy object without bending at the knees causes you to use your back instead of your legs, resulting in back pain.

Lifting places the greatest load on your lower back, and

therefore poses the highest risk of injury. Using proper lifting techniques and correct posture are both critical to prevent injury to your back. How you lift a load is more important than the weight of the load. To help prevent a back injury when lifting follow these tips:

1. Place the load in front of you.
2. Bend the knees to a full squat.
3. Bring the load close to your chest
4. Keep your spine in a neutral position.
5. Tighten the lower back and buttock muscles.
6. Lift with your legs.

Avoid:

1. Lifting from a twisted or sideways position
2. Lifting from a stooped or forward position

Sitting or standing for long periods of time may cause the muscles that support the spine to tighten and cause back pain. After one to two hours, take a postural break.

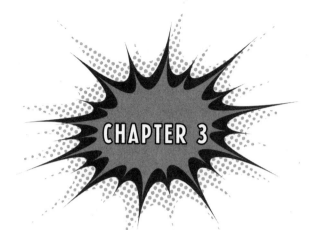

CHAPTER 3

Get Off the Couch!
Too Much Sitting Can
Cause Back Pain

Mother Knows Best—Sit Up Straight!

TIPS FOR SITTING

When we are sitting at a desk or at home on the sofa, we need to use good body mechanics. This must be done at all times. For desk work, consider investing in an ergonomically enhanced chair.

When sitting, always do the following:

- Sit with your buttocks at the back of the seat while maintaining a small space between the back of your knees and the seat of the chair.
- Keep your feet flat on the floor with your knees level with your hips.
- Pull your shoulders back and lift your chest.
- Lift your chin until it is level and relax your jaw.

If your chair has armrests, make sure they are positioned to support the weight of your arms; not too high to make you hunch over or too low to make you reach.

When sitting, footrests can be used to help you maintain good posture. The footrest should be positioned so that your knees are bent comfortably and are level with your hips.

When sitting for a prolonged period, look for a chair that has adjustable lumbar support. If the chair does not have lumbar support, you can increase the support by using a lumbar roll. You can roll up a towel, if you do not have a lumbar roll.

Sitting in the "correct" position for long periods of time will eventually become uncomfortable. After sitting for approximately one to two hours, take a break. Stretching and moving around will help to reduce the stress on your spine. This will also help to prevent muscle fatigue and stiffness. Remember to take a break after driving as well. Too often, people continue to drive long distances without taking a break.

Yes, even when you sleep, you have to do it right to avoid back pain.

CASE HISTORY

Megan is a 35-year-old female who came to the Spine and Orthopedic Pain Center with a need for help with reoccurring lower back pain. With each occurrence, she could hardly walk without experiencing excruciating pain. She rated her pain as 10/10. Megan works as a secretary and sits at a desk all day. She has no leg pain or tingling and has good control of her bowel and bladder. She had no history of trauma or any injury.

On her examination, she had *trigger points* (tender, palpable nodules) in her lower back muscles and decreased range of motion of her back. She did not have any weakness in her legs. Her core was very weak (muscles that stabilize and support the spine).

After a trigger point injection in her lower back muscles (an injection using a local anesthetic, a numbing medication, with a small amount of steroid) was injected into her tender muscle points, she felt better.

She was treated in physical therapy with *myofascial release*, a hands-on technique where the therapist treats the tissues that surround and support the muscles. This helps to restore normal muscle function and increase range of motion.

In therapy, she learned strategies and exercises to help her prevent future reoccurrences of back pain. She was taught what she had been doing wrong. She was instructed not to sit over 1.5 hours without taking a break. Emphasis was placed on how to correct her posture to avoid recurrent back pain.

Megan was given exercises to strengthen her core to take the pressure off her lower back and to increase the flexibility of her back and leg muscles as well. After five weeks, she progressed and was pain-free and using the tools to help **prevent further back pain!**

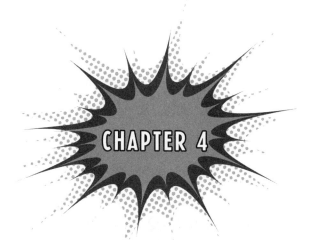

CHAPTER 4

What Can You Do about a Low Back Strain?

WHAT CAUSES LOW BACK STRAINS?

Low back strains are a common cause of low back pain. They occur when muscles are overstretched or torn; when a sudden force, pull, or twist is applied to the muscles in the back, resulting in pain. Most episodes of acute low back pain are caused by damage to the muscles and/or ligaments in the low back. They are the cause of many emergency room visits each year. There are two common types of lower back strain:

1. A **muscle strain** occurs when the muscle is overstretched or torn, resulting in damage to the muscle fibers.
2. A **lumbar sprain** occurs when ligaments are stretched too far or torn. Ligaments are very tough, fibrous-connecting tissues that connect bones together.

WHAT ARE LIGAMENTOUS OR LUMBAR SPRAINS AND WHAT CAUSES THEM?

Lumbar sprains are another common cause of back pain. They occur when the ligaments holding the bones together are torn from their attachments. Sprains happen with quick, unexpected movements. (See above under "Back Strains.")

If it is a muscle strain or a ligament sprain that is causing your pain, the treatment and prognosis for both are the same. Therefore, I will discuss these conditions together.

When the muscles or ligaments in the back are strained or torn, the area around the muscles will usually become inflamed. This inflammation causes the back to spasm. Back spasms can cause severe back pain and restricted movements.

Muscle strains can be caused by any type of movement that puts extra stress on the lower back. Frequent causes include lifting a heavy object, lifting while twisting, or a sudden movement or fall. Pulled muscles also occur while playing sports. This can occur with sports that involve twisting, or any types of sudden impact or jarring motions.

WHAT ARE THE SYMPTOMS OF MUSCLE STRAINS AND LUMBAR SPRAINS?

Symptoms of a pulled muscle in the lower back include the following:

- The pain is usually localized in the lower back (does not radiate down the leg).
- The lower back may be sore to the touch.
- Pain comes on suddenly.
- There may be accompanying muscle spasms.
- Pain is reduced when resting, and may increase with standing or walking.

Severe back pain may resolve quickly, but a lower level of pain, or intermittent flare-ups of pain, may continue for a few weeks or a couple of months.

HOW IS A SPRAIN OR STRAIN DIAGNOSED?

Mild strains and sprains of the lumbar spine can usually be diagnosed by taking the medical history, by reviewing how the injury occurred, and by the symptoms. An examination by your health-care provider can help to determine if you have a lumbar strain or sprain.

HOW ARE MUSCLE STRAINS AND LUMBAR SPRAINS TREATED?

Muscle strains in the back usually heal with time. Most heal within a few days. Almost all strains resolve within three or four weeks. The large muscles in the low back have a good blood supply that carries nutrients to facilitate healing. Treatment includes:

- **Pain medication** (such as acetaminophen)
- **Anti-inflammatory medication** (such as ibuprofen) to reduce the local pain and inflammation. *Avoid* these if you are on blood thinners, have kidney disease, GI conditions, or cardiovascular problems.
- **Muscle relaxants** may be prescribed on a short-term basis to relieve severe lower back pain associated with muscle spasms. These commonly cause drowsiness, so I recommend them at night.
- **Massage** can help promote blood flow in the lower back. This helps with healing, loosens tight lower back muscles, and releases endorphins, the body's natural painkillers.

- **Physical therapy or chiropractic treatment**—gentle manual manipulation—can be done to help loosen tight back muscles and promote healing in the lower back.
- **Ice** can help reduce inflammation. Use it initially. It works well for muscle spasms.
- **Heat therapy** applied to the lower back is helpful longer term to stimulate blood flow and to help heal the injured area. Do not use heat initially.

If the low back pain lasts for more than two weeks, the muscles may start to weaken. Using the lower back muscles is painful;therefore, the tendency is to avoid using them. However, this lack of activity leads to muscle wasting and can cause subsequent weakening. This results in more low back pain because the muscles are not able to help support the spine.

People who are active and well conditioned are much less likely to suffer from low back pain due to muscle strain because regular exercise stretches the muscles. This reduces the risk of muscle tears, strains or spasms.

The spine is supported by three muscles:

1. Extensors (back muscles and gluteal [buttocks] muscles)
2. Flexors (abdominal muscles and iliopsoas [hip flexor] muscles)

3. Obliques or rotators (side muscles)

Although some of these muscles are used in everyday activities, most of them do not get adequate exercise from daily activities. This causes them to weaken with age unless they are specifically exercised. This is why treatment with a physical therapist is helpful in reducing back pain. (See chapter 12 on reducing back pain with physical therapy.)

The hamstring muscle runs through the back of your thigh. Tightness in this muscle limits motion in the pelvis, which can strain the lower back. Therefore, regular hamstring stretching can gradually lengthen these muscles and reduce the stress felt in the lower back. (See the exercises to knock out pain in the back of the book. I have illustrated two ways to stretch your hamstrings.)

Gardening is a hobby of mine, although I don't get to do it as often as I would like. However, over the years, I have learned ten tips for gardening that will help you keep your back in good shape through the spring and summer. The biggest mistake people make when working in the yard is not warming up their muscles prior to starting this activity. It is important to warm up your muscles to prepare for the repetitive movements and heavy lifting required for gardening. I tell my neighbors and friends this every spring when they call about their aches and pains after working in their yards. Yet, every spring, they rush to prune their flowers, clean the beds, and do other yard work without doing warm-ups. Yes, they get backaches.

Remember these tips when doing yard work or gardening:

1. Shoe wear – Yard work can put a lot of strain on your feet and legs. Good foot and arch supports can stop some of that strain from affecting your back. Sandals and flip flops are for the *beach,* not for yard work.

2. Warm Up – Before beginning the tasks, take a few minutes to warm up your muscles by doing some warm-up exercises. These include walking around the yard briskly for a few minutes or doing jumping jacks. Do a few back and hamstring stretches as well. (See illustration at back of book)

3. Drink Lots of Water – Yard work can be exhausting. Therefore, you need adequate water levels to help prevent muscle cramps or spasms and to help prevent dehydration. Muscles need water to function at their best. This allows your muscles to work efficiently with better coordination and to support your physical activity.

4. Variation— Change your gardening tasks. Do a little pruning, raking, and mulching. Avoid performing any particular activity for a prolonged period.

5. Avoid bending – When weeding or doing other activities, avoid bending at the waist for prolonged periods. Repetitive bending will increase the likelihood that your muscles will ache. Kneel or sit on a stool. This will reduce the stress to your back. Keep your gardening tools close at hand.

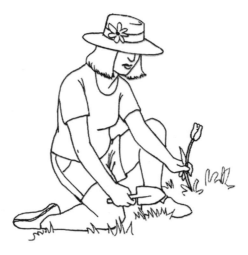

6. Avoid leaning – When mowing, avoid leaning forward as you push the lawn mower. This can strain your back. Be sure to maintain proper posture and push with your arms and legs instead of your back.

7. Lifting – When lifting bags, keep your back straight and bend with your knees. Lift with your legs. Avoid bending at the waist. Make the piles of debris small to decrease the weight. See illustration on page 111 .

8. Avoid Twisting – When raking, avoid twisting your back and stand with your feet shoulder-width apart, one foot in front of the other. Try to keep your back straight.

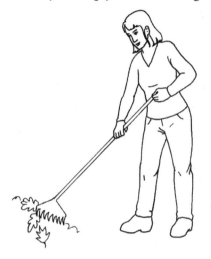

9. Take breaks – Taking a postural break make it less likely that injuries will occur.

10. Ice – Use ice for sore muscles. Ice will decrease muscle spasms.

I hope this helps. Write me at info@knockoutpain.com and let me know if these tips were useful.

What if you follow all of these tips and still have low back pain? I recommend:

- Ice treatments (Ice a little more often).

- Stretching techniques or treatment by a physical thera-pist to help repair and strengthen muscles.

- Lifestyle changes such as weight loss and regular exercise.

CASE HISTORY

During the summer, I saw a 25-year-old female who presented with severe low-back pain after working in her garden. She had significant spasms in her lower back and had difficulty with movements of her back and with standing. She rated her pain as 8 on the scale 0 to 10. Because of her pain, Karen was unable to perform her activities of daily living.

When she came to my office, she had tenderness to palpation in her lower back muscles and decreased range of motion of her back. She did not have any weakness, numbness, or tingling in her legs; no history of bowel or bladder problems. Her core (muscles that stabilize the spine) were very weak.

She was treated in physical therapy with *myofascial release* (a technique where the therapist stretches the muscles using his or her hands). While in therapy, she underwent spinal stabilization training to strengthen her core.

Initially, she was treated with an anti-inflammatory medication. After physical therapy, she was not on any medication for pain, and she was doing well. Ice was used to reduce her spasms.

She now understands the importance of performing her

exercises on a routine basis to maintain the strength of her core. The importance of maintaining strong muscles to support the spine was emphasized. Karen was also instructed on how to maintain proper posture while performing her activities of daily living.

CHAPTER 5

Degenerative Discs Are Another Cause of Back Pain

WHAT IS DEGENERATIVE DISC DISEASE AND WHAT CAUSES IT?

Discs act as cushions between the vertebrae in your spine. As we age, these discs can become thinner, thereby losing some of their shock-absorbing capacity. They also become thinner as they dehydrate. When all that happens, the discs change from a state that allows fluid movement to a stiff and rigid state that restricts your movement and causes pain.

Degenerative disc disease is one of the most common causes

of low back pain and also one of the most misunderstood. Degenerative disc disease (DDD) is typically associated with aging.

WHO GETS IT?

As you age, your discs, like other joints in the body, can *degenerate* (break down) and become problematic: that's a natural part of growing older as your body deals with years of strain, overuse, and maybe even misuse. However, DDD can occur in people as young as 20 years old. In fact, some people may inherit a prematurely aging spine.

Degenerative disc disease involves the intervertebral discs. These are the cushions between your vertebrae in your spine. As you age, the discs can lose flexibility, elasticity, and shock-absorbing characteristics. Between the ages of 25 and 60, the disc spaces begin to lose fluid, and as a result, the disc may experience some fraying and loss of height. If the outer portion of the disc experiences irritation from these issues, it may hurt. The only part of the disc that contains nerve endings and is able to feel pain is the outer portion, which is called the *annulus fibrosus*. Think of this part as being a fibrous ring. The inner portion is filled with a gelatinous substance and is called the *Nucleus pulposus*.

WHAT ARE THE SYMPTOMS OF DEGENERATIVE DISC DISEASE?

If you have chronic back pain (pain that has lasted more than three months), you may have degenerative disc disease. The most frequent symptoms are lower-back pain and spasms. The pain is made worse by sitting, bending, or standing, and is often relieved by lying down. It commonly occurs in your low back (lumbar spine).

HOW IS DEGENERATIVE DISC DISEASE DIAGNOSED?

Diagnostic tests such as an MRI are helpful in identifying areas of disc degeneration.

If conservative treatment fails, a discogram can help to identify problematic discs. A *discogram* is a test used to determine if one or more discs between the bones of the spine are the source of your pain. Using a needle, a special dye is injected into the discs to look at the disc structure in more detail. The test is done under fluoroscopy (a type of low-dose X-ray).

The results are then used to determine if a more advanced treatment is right for you. The discogram is not a treatment for pain and should not be done unless you are seriously considering surgery or similar treatment(s).

Some degenerative discs do not cause pain. However, if the

discs causing the patient's pain are noted during the discogram, surgery can be performed to remove the damaged disc (see discussion under "When Should Surgery Be Done?").

HOW IS DEGENERATIVE DISC DISEASE TREATED?

Nonsurgical Options

Initial treatment is nonsurgical. Your physician may initially prescribe an anti-inflammatory medication and physical therapy to treat degenerative disc disease. A tailored program of physical therapy with spinal stabilization training usually works well for this condition. For some patients, a trial with a narcotic medication might be needed.

Further treatment depends on whether the damaged disc has resulted in other conditions, such as a herniated disc or spinal stenosis. In these cases, an epidural steroid injection can be very effective in resolving the pain. If arthritis in the small joints of the back is the primary problem, injections into these small joints, called facet injections, can be done to relieve pain.

If you suffer from degenerative disc disease, the good news is that this condition usually improves with the appropriate conservative management. The nonsurgical options for treating degenerative disc disease include:

1. Physical therapy
2. Interventional pain management
3. Pain medications
4. Using a semirigid back brace

Nonsurgical treatment is successful over 75% of the time, and patients are often able to avoid surgery. If you have tried nonsurgical treatment for over six months, and the pain is still unbearable, it may be time to start considering surgery. Some people take a longer period of time before they get relief. Undergoing surgery should not be taken lightly.

WHEN SHOULD SURGERY BE DONE?

Deciding whether or not to undergo surgery for degenerative disc disease is an elective decision.

If you have one specific disc that is producing your pain as is shown on the discogram, and all imaging studies (MRI, etc.) point to that same disc as having significant degeneration, then surgery may have a high level of success. But this is not always the case.

Sometimes, even if a technically perfect surgery is performed, the patient may still end up experiencing pain. Surgery is not usually successful in getting rid of all of a patient's back pain. Generally, one should expect to have about a 50 to 75%

reduction in pain with a fusion of a one-level degenerative disc if the surgery is performed successfully.

There are two surgical options for a degenerative disc disease: One is to perform a spinal fusion; the second is to provide an artificial disc replacement. The FDA approved artificial disc replacements over ten years ago.

However, artificial disc replacement surgery has not been shown to be superior to spinal fusions. The success rate is approximately 70%. Therefore, patients should think long and hard prior to undergoing surgical intervention for a degenerative disc. Patients will need physical therapy after surgery, and it can take up to one year before they fully recover from a lumbar fusion.

To give you an idea of how you will feel after a fusion, ask your doctor to prescribe a rigid back brace prior to undergoing surgery. If you tolerate the brace and it relieves your pain, this might be a good indication that you will get some relief from a lumbar fusion.

CASE HISTORY

Bob is a 68-year-old gentleman with a history of degenerative disc disease. His MRI of the lumbar spine demonstrates degenerative disc disease at multiple levels. He does not want surgery, and he came to me to explore other options. He had no weakness of his lower extremities and no loss of control of his bowel or bladder.

He started a trial of physical therapy and was taught how to strengthen his core with lumbar stabilization training. He also learned stretches to keep his hips flexible. Bob did abdominal strengthening and was treated with manual therapy as well. He was given a customized home exercise program.

During therapy, it was discovered that Bob was not wearing supportive shoes. After learning about the biomechanics of the spine, how to perform lumbar stabilization exercises, and with the use of proper shoe wear, Bob has done well over the past two years. He is happy that he was able to learn what he could do to avoid undergoing the knife as a means of relieving his pain. He was given a semirigid back brace to use *only* when he performs lifting activities because you should never wear a back brace all day long. We want you to keep your muscles strong; therefore, you must use them.

CHAPTER 6

Is Your Pain From a Herniated Disc?

WHAT IS A HERNIATED (RUPTURED) DISC AND WHAT CAUSES IT?

When you experience back pain that shoots down your leg, everyday activities become difficult or intolerable. Ending the pain becomes increasingly important. One cause of back pain that shoots down your leg is a **herniated disc**, sometimes called a **ruptured disc**.

Your spine is made up of bones **(vertebrae)** cushioned by small pads of cartilage and by discs consisting of a tough, outer layer (**annulus**) and a soft, inner jelly layer (**nucleus pulposus**).

When a herniated disc occurs in your back, a small portion of the nucleus pulposus pushes out, or ruptures, through a tear in the annulus into the spinal canal. This can irritate a nerve and result in pain, numbness, or weakness in your leg or foot. When this happens, a condition we commonly refer to as *sciatica* occurs. This results when the herniated disc presses on the main nerve that travels down your leg and causes pain to radiate from the buttock down the back of the leg.

SYMPTOMS

The most **common signs and symptoms** of a herniated disc are:

- **Sciatica — a radiating, aching pain** that sometimes includes tingling and numbness that starts in your buttocks and extends down the back or side of one leg
- **Pain, numbness or weakness** in one leg
- **Low back pain or leg pain that worsens** when you sit, cough, or sneeze

You need to seek prompt medical attention if:

- You lose control of your bladder or bowels

- You develop increased numbness or weakness in one or both legs
- You experience back pain that is disabling for several days

DIAGNOSIS

You can have a herniated disc without knowing it. Herniated discs sometimes are visible on the MRIs of people who have no symptoms of a disc problem. Just because you have a herniated disc on your MRI does not mean that disc is causing your pain. That's why it is important for your physician to talk with you and examine you to determine if your MRI findings correlate with your history and physical examination. Otherwise, you could undergo surgery for a disc that was not causing your pain. To **accurately diagnose** a herniated disc, your physician should perform a thorough evaluation that may include tests such as an MRI, CT scan, or Nerve Conduction/EMG.

TREATMENT: YOU DON'T HAVE TO UNDERGO SURGERY FOR A HERNIATED DISC

A herniated disc generally gets better with conservative treatment. Therefore, surgery for a herniated disc is usually not necessary. Approximately 90% of patients with herniated discs can be treated without surgery.

However, when the pain from the disc continues, an epidural steroid injection using X-ray guidance can be helpful. During this procedure, an anti-inflammatory medication is injected around the inflamed disc and nerves to decrease the pain and irritation.

Physical therapy is important for nearly everyone who suffers with disc disease. Physical therapists teach you how to properly lift, dress, walk, sit, and perform other daily activities to reduce back and leg pain when the herniation is in the back (lumbar spine). Additionally, a therapist will teach you the most effective exercises to strengthen the muscles that help to support the spine. In physical therapy, you will also learn how to increase the flexibility in your spine and legs or arms. Remember, with appropriate treatment, 90% of patients with a herniated disc can be treated with nonsurgically.

During surgery for a herniated disc, the surgeon usually makes a small incision in the back and removes a portion of the disc that is pressing on the nerve. The whole disc is not removed. However, if you continue to use poor body mechanics and lift something incorrectly or engage in poor and prolonged sitting, more disc material can squirt out, even after surgery. This is why surgery does not cure problems due to disc herniations. Ultimately, it is up to you to use correct body mechanics of the spine to help prevent recurrent disc herniations.

WHAT IS A DISC? (REVISITED)

It is important that you clearly understand what a disc is. For those of you who didn't understand what I said at the beginning of the chapter, I will explain it another way.

The disc sits between the bones in the spine and provides cushioning as well as connecting one bone to the other. It is the natural shock absorber in your spine. The disc is somewhat similar to a tire in that it has a rubbery layer around the outside called the *annulus fibrosus*. The inside of the disc is filled with a gelatinous-like substance called the *nucleus pulposus*.

When the disc *herniates*, the outer covering of the disc, the annulus fibrosus, breaks. This allows the inside material, the nucleus pulposus, to squirt out. When this material squirts out, it can rest against the nerves as the nerves leave your spine. This results in back and leg pain. When this material—the nucleus pulposus—is on your nerves, the pressure it exerts on the nerves can sometimes become so great that there can be loss of nerve function. When the nerve function is lost or diminished, you experience numbness or weakness.

A disc can also be thought of as a sponge—a sponge that is

filled with water. When a disc becomes very, very inflamed it is like a big and swollen sponge. When it is big like this and pressing on the nerve, it causes pain, usually down your leg. However, if that sponge sits on your sink for a while, what happens? It usually dries out. This is the same process that happens with the disc. The disc naturally dries out, or the body reabsorbs the disc material over time. As it dries out just like a sponge, it shrinks, which causes less pressure on the nerve.

If that is the case, you might ask, why does one need surgery for a disc herniation? The natural process is that a disc will dry out over time. But what happens if you have poor body mechanics? You can go through recurrent cycles where more disc material is squirted out again and again.

Think of your nerve as being like a toothbrush. The gelatinous material inside the disc is the toothpaste. When that toothpaste squirts out on the toothbrush, it causes numbness, tingling, and weakness. Anti-inflammatory medications can help to calm down the irritation. Likewise, an injection of a small amount of steroid around the nerves exactly where the problem is —for example, an epidural steroid injection—helps calm down the inflammation while the body's natural processes work to reabsorb the material from the disc. This is also why surgery does not cure the problem.

CASE HISTORY

Several months ago, I saw a 45-year-old male who injured himself while working at a construction site. Jack injured his back while lifting a fifty-pound box filled with floor tile. He came to see me after he developed severe back pain with mild weakness, numbness, and tingling in the left leg. He had no change in his bowel or bladder function. Jack could barely sit down when I saw him. He was unable to work and described his pain as excruciating, rating it as a 10 out of 10 on a scale of 0 to 10, with 10 being the worst possible pain. His pain increased with coughing and sneezing.

Like Jack, whenever you experience back pain that shoots down your leg, everyday activities become difficult or intolerable. Resolving the pain becomes increasingly important. One cause of back pain that shoots down your leg is a herniated disc, sometimes called a ruptured disc, or commonly referred to as "sciatica."

Jack had an MRI, which revealed a large, herniated disc.

I performed two epidural injections. The first one gave him 50% relief, and the second one gave him an additional 30% relief. He also had a short trial of physical therapy focusing on reducing his pain while teaching him how to perform his activities of daily living pain-free.

Therapy was key to Jack's rehabilitation since the ability to lift and carry heavy objects was an important part of his work responsibilities. His therapy focused on improving his core strength and his ability to perform his specific work tasks.

I cannot stress enough that physical therapy is important for nearly everyone who suffers with disc disease. Physical therapists teach you how to properly lift, dress, walk, sit, and perform other daily activities to reduce back and leg pain when the herniation is in the back (lumbar spine). They can also demonstrate proper postural recommendations to relieve the pain from herniations. Additionally, a therapist can teach you the most effective exercises to strengthen the muscles that help support the spine. In physical therapy, you will also learn how to increase the flexibility in your spine and legs.

Today, I'm happy to report that Jack is doing well, back to working full-time without any symptoms of back pain or weakness, numbness, or tingling in the left leg.

Remember, 90% of patients with a herniated disc can be appropriately treated nonsurgically. Just because a disc is large, it doesn't mean you have to undergo surgery.

This is why it is so important to learn the 12 steps to prevent back pain discussed in chapter 16.

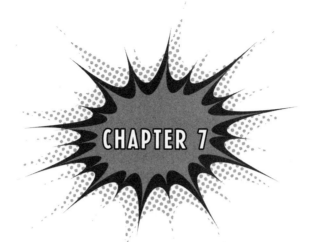

CHAPTER 7

Spinal Stenosis:
How to Live With It

WHAT IS SPINAL STENOSIS AND WHAT CAUSES IT?

Spinal stenosis also causes back pain. Spinal stenosis usually occurs after the age of 50, when arthritis in the spine can lead to a narrowing of areas in the lumbar (back) or cervical (neck) spine, which compresses nerves within the canal, causing pressure on the spinal cord or one or more of the spinal nerves. The compression of the nerves can lead to pain and numbness in the legs and may cause the pain you are experiencing.

Spinal stenosis may be caused by:

- Arthritis involving the spine, usually in middle-aged or elderly people
- Herniated or slipped disc, two different types of disc problems
- Injury that causes pressure on the nerve roots or the spinal cord itself
- Defect in the spine that was present at birth (congenital defect)
- Tumors in the spine

SYMPTOMS

The narrowing of the spinal canal can result in a number of **symptoms**. However, patients begin to experience problems when inflammation of the nerves occurs at levels of increased pressure.

Often, symptoms will gradually worsen over time and can include:

- Numbness, tingling, cramping, or pain in the back, buttocks, thighs, or calves
- Weakness of a portion of a leg

Symptoms are more likely to be present or get worse when

you stand or walk upright. They will often lessen or disappear when you sit down or lean forward. Most people with spinal stenosis cannot walk for a long periods of time.

Symptoms that are more serious include:

- Difficulty or imbalance when walking
- Problems controlling urine or bowel movements

DIAGNOSIS

The diagnosis begins with a thorough medical history and physical examination, with diagnostic testing including X-rays, MRI, and/or CT scans to identify the source of the pain.

TREATMENT: THREE OPTIONS TO AVOID SURGERY IF YOU HAVE SPINAL STENOSIS

Hundreds of thousands of back surgeries are performed every year in the United States. However, if you struggle with spinal stenosis, you may find relief and avoid surgery. Spinal stenosis responds well to nonsurgical treatment. In many cases, surgery in spinal stenosis can be avoided and the pain can be eliminated! Medications, physical therapy, and epidural injections are viable nonsurgical options for treating spinal stenosis.

Pain can be relieved with various medications depending upon your symptoms. Often, *narcotics* are not prescribed to treat the pain from spinal stenosis.

An individualized physical therapy program can be very helpful. Physical therapy can help patients learn how to take care of their backs and how to manage recurrent episodes of back pain, thereby reducing the need for medications in most cases. In physical therapy, the muscles of the abdomen, back, and legs are strengthened, which helps reduce the symptoms of nerve compression. Education on proper posture and body mechanics are an essential part of this process, thereby helping to avoid surgery.

When pain is not relieved by medications or physical therapy, an epidural steroid injection (ESI) can be performed under fluoroscopy for symptomatic relief. Fluoroscopic or X-ray guidance is the current standard of care with epidural steroid injections. Multiple studies have shown that the injection is improperly placed up to 34% of the time outside the epidural space when fluoroscopy is not used.

An epidural can help to further reduce pain and inflammation by reducing compression on the nerves. Usually, you will notice a difference within 48 to 72 hours. If the pain is persistent and does not respond to nonsurgical measures, surgery may be necessary to try to improve your quality of life. In these cases, surgery is considered an elective procedure.

However, if spinal stenosis is causing a worsening neurologic deficit, such as a foot drop, surgery may be indicated and not elective. In rare cases, some patients experience problems controlling urine or bowel movements because of stenosis. If you find yourself in this position, you should definitely undergo a surgical evaluation.

In severe cases of stenosis, surgery is performed. The goal of the surgery is to relieve pressure on the spinal cord or spinal nerve by widening the spinal canal or the foraminal canal. This is done by removing, trimming, or realigning the abnormal anatomy that is causing the compression of the nerves. However, before undergoing surgery, ask your doctor if you are a candidate for a nonsurgical treatment to relieve your pain from spinal stenosis.

CASE HISTORY

Mark has been a patient of mine for ten years. Ten years ago, he was diagnosed with severe spinal stenosis and told that he needed to have surgery. His primary care provider referred him to me for a second opinion.

When he came to my office to be examined, he was complaining of excruciating pain that radiated from his back down to both legs. On a scale of 1-10, his pain was 10. He had no lower extremity weakness or loss of control of his bowel or bladder. However, his pain increased with walking and was relieved with sitting.

The MRI of his lumbar spine confirmed that he had spinal stenosis. Mark was very active and he did not want surgery. Therefore, I recommended that we try a conservative approach to relieve his pain and increase his function.

Initially, I gave him a couple of epidural injections that provided considerable relief. Later, Mark was started on a trial of physical therapy. As was the case for my other patients, a customized physical therapy program was recommended for him based on his diagnosis. In physical therapy, he was taught specific exercises to treat spinal stenosis.

During therapy, he learned that his exercise program had to be specific for his diagnosis. It was important that Mark perform all of his exercises with his spine in a neutral position. It was equally important that he keep his spine in a neutral position while performing his activities of daily living.

Today, Mark continues to remain pain-free. He has no pain in his back and legs. He rarely takes any medication for pain, and he was never treated with narcotics. Mark remains active; he has always been an active person because he is a football coach.

Mark continues to play golf and does his yard work without any pain. He performs the exercises he learned in physical therapy on a routine basis. To avoid recurrent back pain and to ensure that he remains stable without leg weakness, Mark follows up with me twice a year.

FREQUENTLY ASKED QUESTIONS ABOUT SPINAL STENOSIS

Do your legs or back feel better when you are leaning over a shopping cart when walking? If so, you might have spinal stenosis.

What Is Spinal Stenosis?

Spinal stenosis is a narrowing of areas in the lumbar (back) or cervical (neck) spine that causes pressure on the spinal cord or one or more of the spinal nerves.

Who Gets Spinal Stenosis?

Spinal stenosis is most common in men and women over 50 years of age. However, it may occur in younger people who are born with a narrowing of the spinal canal or who suffer an injury to the spine.

What Causes Spinal Stenosis?

Narrowing of the spinal canal leads to spinal stenosis. It can result from congenital conditions or be acquired.

When people are born with a small spinal canal, it is a condition called *congenital spinal stenosis.* Sometimes people have a curvature of the spine known as *scoliosis,* which can put pressure on nerves. Either of these conditions can lead to spinal stenosis.

Acquired conditions can also cause spinal stenosis. The most common cause of spinal stenosis results from a degenerative process that is part of aging. As you age, your spinal structures change. Ligaments may thicken; bones and joints may also enlarge due to wear and tear over time, and spinal stenosis can occur.

When one vertebrae slips forward on the one below it, a condition called *spondylolisthesis* results. This slippage can also result in spinal stenosis.

Spinal stenosis can also occur because of tumors in the spine.

Any of these processes can cause narrowing of the spinal canal, resulting in spinal stenosis.

What Are the Symptoms of Spinal Stenosis?

Narrowing of the spinal canal can cause a number of symptoms. People often experience numbness, weakness, tingling, cramping, or pain in the back, buttocks, thighs, and calves.

Symptoms from spinal stenosis are more likely to be present or get worse when you stand or walk upright. However, symptoms often disappear or lessen with sitting or flexing the lower back. You may notice that you feel better when you walk with a grocery cart; this is because the back is placed in a flexed position.

With more severe stenosis, people may have problems with bowel and bladder functions and weakness of the foot.

Cauda equina syndrome is a very severe and rare condition. It is caused by severe narrowing of the spinal canal that compresses the nerve roots below the level of the spinal cord. With cauda equina syndrome, symptoms can include loss of control of the bowel and bladder functions and lower extremity weakness, accompanied by loss of feeling in one or both legs. One may also experience numbness in the groin or in the area of contact if you were sitting in a saddle. Cauda equina syndrome is considered a surgical emergency.

How Is Spinal Stenosis Diagnosed?

The diagnosis begins with a thorough medical history and physical examination. Diagnostic testing, including X-rays, MRIs, and/or CT scans can be done to identify the source of pain.

What Are Treatment Options for Spinal Stenosis?

Nonsurgical options are usually prescribed for treatment of spinal stenosis unless the person has severe or progressive nerve damage.

Medications such as nonsteroidal anti-inflammatory drugs like Ibuprofen and Naproxen can be prescribed to reduce pain and inflammation. Ask your physician before taking an anti-infammatory medication.

Epidural steroid injections can be prescribed for pain relief. These injections are also a very good option for those who are unable to undergo surgery because of other medical problems.

Physical therapy can be a viable option to help maintain the motion of the spine and to strengthen abdominal and back muscles. Aquatic or water therapy is also an excellent option for persons with spinal stenosis.

When Should Surgery Be Done?

Nonsurgical treatment is done initially to determine if it helps reduce the symptoms from spinal stenosis. However, surgery might be performed immediately when a patient has leg weakness and impaired bowel or bladder function. The effectiveness of nonsurgical treatments and the severity of the patient's pain will all play a part in determining whether or not to have spinal surgery.

The goal of surgery is to relieve pressure on the spinal cord or nerves and to restore and maintain alignment and strength of the spine.

Consult your physician if you have symptoms of spinal stenosis.

CHAPTER 8

Do You Have a Slipped Disc?

WHAT IS SPONDYLOLISTHESIS?

Spondylolisthesis (slipped disc) is a condition where a vertebra in the spine slips out of place, causing pain. When one vertebra slips forward over the one beneath it, the spinal canal becomes narrower. With less room to function in their natural positions, the spinal cord and nerves become irritated and inflamed, which causes painful symptoms.

WHO GETS SPONDYLOLISTHESIS?

Spondylolisthesis is a fairly common cause of lower back pain and leg pain in younger adults (ages 30 to 50). Degenerative spondylolisthesis is a fairly common cause of pain in older adults (ages 50 and up). The most common symptoms are lower back pain and/or leg pain.

WHAT CAUSES SPONDYLOLISTHESIS?

Spondylolisthesis can be caused by:
  A. Birth defect
  B. Fractures
  C. Overuse
  D. Degeneration due to age
  E. Tumors
  F. Surgery

WHAT ARE THE SYMPTOMS OF SPONDYLOLISTHESIS?

The symptoms of degenerative spondylolisthesis are very commonly the same as that of spinal stenosis. The main symptoms of degenerative spondylolisthesis include low back pain and/or leg pain. However, some patients do not have any back pain with degenerative spondylolisthesis, and others have primarily back pain and no leg pain. Sometimes, people often complain of an aching in one or both legs, or a tired feeling down the legs when they stand for a prolonged period of time or try to walk any distance.

Most patients do not have a lot of pain while sitting. When we sit, the spinal canal is more open. However, in the upright position, the spinal canal gets smaller, making the stenosis worse and pinching the nerve roots in the canal. Most people have pain with extension (that is, when they arch the back backwards). When the nerve root is pinched, one can have weakness in the legs, but true nerve root damage is rare.

HOW IS SPONDYLOLISTHESIS DIAGNOSED?

A thorough physical examination is the first step in diagnosing this condition. X-rays of the lumbar (lower) spine are crucial for determining whether a vertebra is out of place. Sometimes, your physician may order a computerized tomography (CT) scan if the misplaced bone is pressing on your nerves.

WHAT ARE TREATMENT OPTIONS FOR SPONDYLOLISTHESIS?

Nonsurgical treatment options include:

- **Pain medications**
- **Activity modification**—spend more time sitting and

less time standing or walking. Avoid standing or walking for long periods. Also avoid activities that require bending backward.

- The use of **cold packs and/or moist heating pads** might be helpful.
- Using a stationary bicycle because activities in the sitting position are usually well tolerated.
- Another option is **aquatic therapy** – physical therapy done while in a pool. In the pool, water provides support and you can exercise in a flexed- forward position.
- **Physical therapy with manual manipulation** by appropriately trained health professionals can help reduce pain by mobilizing painful, dysfunctional joints.
- **Epidural injections**

If you have severe pain, especially leg pain, epidural steroid injections may be beneficial. These injections are effective in helping to reduce the pain and inflammation. They can increase a patient's function up to 50% of the time. An epidural steroid injection can be done up to three times per year. The length of time that the lumbar epidural injection is effective varies.

Bracing—A semirigid back brace helps with lifting and repetitive activities. Never use the brace all day. We want to keep your back muscles strong.

WHEN SHOULD SURGERY BE CONSIDERED?

If you have no relief from conservative management, and your pain is disabling, surgery can be considered. Surgery is also indicated when the patient experiences progressive neurologic deficits (weakness of the legs or loss of control of bladder or bowel function).

Surgery is done to realign the slipped vertebrae to alleviate pressure on the nerve and provide stability of the spine. Surgery for a degenerative spondylolisthesis usually includes two parts, done together in one operation: A *decompression* (called a *laminectomy*) *and* a *fusion with instrumentation* (usually rods and screws). Decompression surgery, referred to as a *laminectomy alone*, is usually not advisable, as the instability is still present. Therefore, a fusion will be needed in up to 60% of patients.

A fusion is a difficult surgery to recover from, since there is a lot of dissection. A fusion usually involves putting hardware into the spine (rods or screws are typically used). It can take up to a year to fully recover. Usually, most patients can start most of their activities after the fusion has healed for three months. Once the bone is fused, then the more active the patient is, the stronger the bone will become. Usually, the patient will need physical therapy after surgery to facilitate the rehabilitation process.

There are numerous risks and possible complications with surgery for degenerative spondylolisthesis, and they are basically the same as for any fusion surgery. There are risks of nonunion (failed fusion), hardware failure, continued pain, adjacent segment degeneration, infection, bleeding, dural leak, nerve root damage, and all the possible general anesthetic risks (e.g., blood clots, pulmonary emboli, pneumonia, heart attack, or stroke). Most of these complications are rare, but increased risks can be seen in certain situations. Conditions that increase the risks of surgery include smoking (or any nicotine intake), obesity, multilevel fusions, osteoporosis (thinning of the bones), diabetes, rheumatoid arthritis, or prior failed back surgery.

In patients who have multiple medical problems, surgery can be very risky. For some patients, even if nonsurgical treatments have failed to alleviate their symptoms, surgery may present too much of a risk, and periodic epidural injections, combined with activity modification and physical therapy, may be their best option.

After a fusion, degeneration of the spinal segment above or below the fusion is also possible. Years later, another surgery might be required because of the degeneration of this segment.

CASE HISTORY

Joseph is a 30-year-old male who presented with lower back pain, muscle tightness, and stiffness. His pain radiated from his lower back to his buttocks. Sometimes, his pain radiated to both legs. The pain was rated 8/10 (horrible) and increased with standing.

When I saw Joseph, he had decreased range of motion in his lower back, tightness in his back muscles, and tenderness of the muscles in his lower back. He also had tightness of his hamstrings, hip flexors, and muscles of his buttocks.

X-rays of the lumbar spine revealed a mild-to-moderate slippage of the L4 vertebrae over the L5 vertebrae (*spondylolisthesis*). Spondylolistheses are graded from 0 to 4. Zero means no slippage, grade I less than 25% slippage, grade II 25 to 50%, and so on.

Joseph was given pain medication for a short period of time to bring his pain under control. He was treated with physical therapy designed to strengthen his abdominal and back muscles while keeping his spine in a neutral position. It is important to have both strong abdominal and back muscles to support the spine.

It was emphasized to Joseph that he maintain the good posture positions he was taught, and he was also given stretching exercises to increase the flexibility of his muscles in his back and legs.

Joseph was given a semirigid back brace for support with lifting and repetitive activities. The importance of keeping his spine in a neutral position was stressed while performing his activities of daily living. He was told not to wear the brace all day and to perform his exercises daily.

With this program, he was able to avoid having a lumbar fusion (having rods and screws) in his back. Joseph is seen annually in follow-up to monitor his spondylolisthesis.

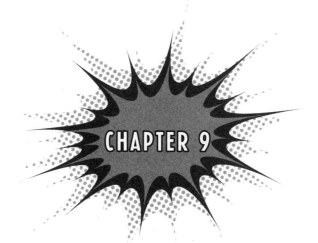

Osteoporosis Affects Both Men and Women

WHAT IS OSTEOPOROSIS?

steoporosis commonly affects the thoracic (midback) and thoracolumbar regions of the spine and may cause debilitating pain. This disorder is caused by a loss of bone mineral density resulting in fragile bones, which can lead to fractures, known as *compression fractures,* which result in very uncomfortable back pain. This can lead to a loss of height, stooped posture, and sometimes a humped back.

WHO GETS OSTEOPOROSIS?

Although it is usually thought of as "a woman's disease," osteoporosis affects both women and men. In fact, in the United States, loss of bone density resulting in osteoporosis affects millions of men, and statistics indicate that 80% of women and 20% of men are affected by osteoporosis. In men, osteoporosis is sometimes attributable to lifestyle habits. These habits can be changed and possibly help avoid the onset of osteoporosis.

According to the National Osteoporosis Foundation, women can lose up to 20% of their bone density in the first five to seven years after menopause. This makes women more susceptible to osteoporosis than men.

WHAT CAUSES OSTEOPOROSIS?

In their 30s, men have accumulated significantly more bone mass than women. However, as both men and women age, bone loss gradually outpaces new bone growth. Following menopause, women lose significantly more bone than men do. By ages 65 to 70, both men and women lose bone mass at the same rate. Therefore, physicians typically watch for signs of osteoporosis once menopause happens.

In men, the most common causes that contribute to osteoporosis include low levels of testosterone, alcohol abuse, smoking, glucocorticoid medications, calcium lost in the urine, and immobilization.

WHAT ARE THE SYMPTOMS OF OSTEOPOROSIS?

In women, the loss of bone mineral density can result in fragile bones, which can lead to fractures, known as *compression fractures*, which result in very uncomfortable back pain. This can lead to a loss of height, stooped posture, and sometimes a humped back.

Osteoporosis is usually only discovered in a man when he goes to see his physician with a complaint of sudden back pain or a fracture. Therefore, men should inform their physicians if they experience a sudden loss in height or a change in posture.

Osteoporosis causes long-term loss of mobility that requires extensive patient care. One in every two women age 50 and older will have an osteoporosis-related fracture, while fractures occur in one in four men. The rate of hip fractures is two to three times higher in women than men. Six months after a hip fracture, only 15 % of hip fracture patients can walk across a room on their own. However, at one year after the fracture, twice as many men die from a hip fracture compared to women.

HOW IS OSTEOPOROSIS DIAGNOSED?

Bone mineral density exams are typically done through X-rays focused on the hip and lower spine (back) regions. These are the areas where fractures and the early signs of osteoporosis manifest as the bones begin to thin from the disease. Like women, men suspected of having osteoporosis are given a medical workup that includes a complete medical history, X-rays, urine and blood tests, and a bone density screening called a *dual-energy X-ray absorptiometry*, or DXA test, that measures bone density at the hip and spine.

WHAT ARE THE TREATMENT OPTIONS FOR OSTEOPOROSIS?

You can control some of the risks for osteoporosis, which include poor diet, smoking, excessive intake of alcohol, and inactivity. The treatment of osteoporosis can include medications, hormone therapy, mineral supplements, physical activity, and recommendations for lifestyle changes.

Things You Can Start to Do Today to Prevent Osteoporosis

- Quit smoking.
- Decrease your alcohol consumption.

- Eat more dairy products such as low-fat milk, yogurt, nonfat dried milk powder, and cheese.
- Choose calcium-fortified cereal, orange juice, and bread.
- Eat more nondairy foods that naturally contain calcium, such as spinach, almonds, and broccoli.
- Eat more food that contains Vitamin D, such as egg yolk, vitamin D fortified dairy products, liver, and saltwater fish.
- Take calcium supplements (if you don't get enough calcium from your diet).
- Start doing resistance exercises like weight lifting (consult with your physician first).
- Start doing weight-bearing exercises like walking, jogging, stair climbing, or dancing (consult with your physician first).
- Talk to your physician about minimizing the intake of medications that can cause bone loss.

CASE HISTORY

Mrs. Smith is a 75-year-old female who presented with moderate chronic thoracic (midback) pain. She had a history of osteoporosis confirmed by a bone density test. Her primary care doctor prescribed medication to treat her osteoporosis.

Mrs. Smith's exam was notable for kyphosis (hump back) of the midback. She also had tenderness to palpation over her thoracic vertebrae.

She was prescribed upper-chest stretches to increase the flexibility in her thoracic spine. She was also given exercises that strengthened her upper back to help maintain an erect posture. Mrs. Smith was encouraged to eat more dairy products and foods that contain Vitamin D.

To prevent osteoporosis, it is important to perform weight-bearing exercises such as walking, stair climbing, and upper-extremity resistance exercises. You should also avoid smoking.

Remember: osteoporosis is not a condition only found in women. I encourage men to get busy protecting your bones as well. Get rid of the cigarettes, eat more dairy foods, and start performing weight-bearing exercises.

CHAPTER 10

How Does Facet Joint Osteoarthritis Cause Low Back Pain?

WHAT IS FACET JOINT OSTEOARTHRITIS AND WHAT CAUSES IT?

*F*acet joint osteoarthritis* occurs when *osteoarthritis* (degenerative arthritis) causes a breakdown of the cartilage between the facet joints (small joints in the back). When the joints move, the lack of cartilage causes pain as well as loss of motion and stiffness. This pain is usually more pronounced first thing in the morning and later in the day.

WHO GETS FACET JOINT OSTEOARTHRITIS?

Facet problems can be caused by a combination of aging, pressure overload of your facet joints, and injury. As the discs degenerate, they wear down and begin to collapse. This narrows the space between each vertebra, which affects the way your facet joints line up. When this occurs, it places too much pressure on the cartilage surface of the facet joint. The excessive pressure leads to damage of the articular surface, and eventually the cartilage begins to wear away. When facet joint arthritis gets bad enough, the cartilage and fluid that lubricate the facet joints are eventually destroyed. This leaves bone rubbing on bone.

WHAT ARE THE SYMPTOMS OF FACET JOINT OSTEOARTHRITIS?

Facet joint disorders are some of the most common of all the recurrent, disabling, low back problems. Lumbar facet joint pain is typically intermittent, generally unpredictable, and occurs a few times per month or per year. Symptoms may include:

- Persistent point tenderness overlying the inflamed facet joints and some degree of loss in the spinal muscle flexibility

- More discomfort while leaning backward
- Radiating pain into the buttocks and down the back of the upper leg.

HOW IS FACET JOINT OSTEOARTHRITIS DIAGNOSED?

Plain X-ray films should be obtained and examined. Usually, the abnormal facet changes can be seen. However, a CT scan can reveal more information about not only the facet joints but also other structures of the spinal segment.

The most definitive diagnosis of facet joint pain can be made by a facet joint injection (or *facet joint block*), which injects the suspicious facet joints with a small volume of a combination of X-ray contrast material, local anesthetic, and cortisone. If the injection relieves the pain, then this helps to identify that the facet is the source of the pain.

WHAT ARE THE TREATMENT OPTIONS FOR FACET JOINT OSTEOARTHRITIS?

To break up a cycle of recurring, acute facet joint pain, a number of treatments can be used successfully. *Nonsurgical treatment options* include:

- Exercises with instructions by a trained physical thera-

pist or chiropractor (see the section on physical therapy
and back pain)

- Improving your posture (see the section on posture)

A very useful exercise when standing or sitting is the poste-
rior pelvic tilt, where one pinches the buttocks and abdominals
and rotates the pelvis backwards. This flexes the lumbar spine.
Hold that position for several seconds, several times per day.

- Moist heat or cold packs may help alleviate painful episodes
- Activity modification, such as shortening or eliminating
  a long daily commute or adding frequent postural breaks
- The use of ant-inflammatory medication, such as Ibuprofen or Naproxen
- Joint manipulation by a physical therapist trained in
  manual techniques or a chiropractor may also provide
  pain relief

WHEN SHOULD SURGERY BE DONE?

Sometimes, lasting relief of the facet joint problem can be obtained by destroying some of the tiny nerve endings serving
the joints. This can be accomplished by performing a *facet rhi-
zotomy*. This is performed under X-ray guidance.

In unusually severe and persistent problems, degeneration of the adjoining disc is nearly always present, so the segment may require a surgery called a *lumbar fusion*. As previously discussed (see chapter 5), one must think long and hard before undergoing a spinal fusion.

For the vast majority of patients, a combination of changes in lifestyle, medications, and proper exercises and posture will reduce the problem to a manageable level and surgery is not needed.

CASE HISTORY

Joanne is a 55-year-old female with a history of facet arthritis. (The *facets* are the small joints in the back.) Her pain was worse with standing and leaning backward. When leaning backward, her pain radiated from her back to her buttocks.

She was given an injection into her lumbar facets using a numbing medication and a small amount of steroid. This relieved her pain and helped her to participate in physical therapy. Since the injection relieved her pain, this confirmed that her facets were the cause of her pain.

In physical therapy, Joanne was treated with joint mobilizations to increase the motion of her facets.

Emphasis was also placed on modifying her activities to reduce her back pain. She received instructions in a lumbar stabilization program designed to reduce overloading of her facet joints.

Pain from facet joint arthritis can be unpredictable and can occur a few times per month or a few times a year. Therefore, it is important to maintain good posture and to return for follow-up with your spine specialist when a flare-up occurs to help break the cycle of your pain.

CHAPTER 11

Is Your Back Pain due to Sacroiliac (SI) Joint Dysfunction?

WHAT IS SACROILIAC (SI) JOINT DYSFUNCTION?

A painful *sacroiliac (SI) joint* is one of the more common causes of mechanical low back pain. Yet, it is often *not diagnosed*. There are two SI joints, each located on either side of the sacrum in the lower back area. These joints allow twisting movements when we move our legs.

There are many different terms for sacroiliac joint problems, including *SI joint dysfunction, SI joint syndrome, SI joint strain,* and *SI joint inflammation (sacroiliitis).* Each of these terms refers to a condition that causes pain in the SI joints from a variety of causes.

WHAT CAUSES SACROILIAC JOINT DYSFUNCTION?

There are many **different causes** of SI joint pain. The SI joints have a cartilage layer covering the bone that allows for some movement and acts as a shock absorber between the bones. When this cartilage is damaged or worn away, the bones begin to rub on each other, and degenerative arthritis (osteoarthritis) occurs. This is the most common cause of SI joint dysfunction.

Sacroiliac joint dysfunction also may occur when an SI joint is injured or irritated. This is seldom dangerous and rarely requires surgery.

Pregnancy may also be a factor in the development of SI joint problems. During pregnancy, hormones are released that allow ligaments to relax. The relaxation of the ligaments holding the SI joints together allows for increased motion in the joints and can lead to increased stresses and abnormal wear.

SI joint dysfunction can also occur from trauma, such as injuries resulting from a fall or associated with a motor vehicle accident.

Another, less frequent cause is having one leg that is shorter than the other; the abnormal alignment may cause SI joint pain.

SYMPTOMS OF SACROILIAC (SI) JOINT DYSFUNCTION

The most common symptom of SI joint dysfunction is sacroiliac joint pain. Patients often experience pain in the lower back or the back of the hips. Pain may also be present in the groin and thighs. The pain is typically worse with standing and walking and improved when lying down. Inflammation and arthritis in the SI joint can also cause stiffness and a burning sensation in the pelvis.

DIAGNOSIS OF SACROILIAC (SI) JOINT DYSFUNCTION

The diagnosis of sacroiliac joint dysfunction is often overlooked.

The most accurate method of diagnosing SI joint dysfunction is by direct injection into the SI joint, which numbs the irritated area. An anesthetic material with a steroid can be injected directly into the SI joint. This is usually performed with X-ray guidance to verify that the injection is correctly placed in the SI joint. If the anesthetic and steroid relieve the pain from inflammation within the SI joint, this verifies that the SI joint is the source of the pain, and treatment can target the SI joint specifically.

Call your physician to determine if your back pain is due to sacroiliac dysfunction or inflammation of the SI joint.

WHAT ARE THE TREATMENT OPTIONS FOR SACROILIAC (SI) JOINT PAIN?

Oral anti-inflammatory medications (NSAIDs, ibuprofen [Motrin], naproxen [Naprosyn] or others) are often effective in pain relief for SI joint pain.

Additionally, physical therapy can also be very helpful. Pain in the SI joint is often related to either too much motion or not enough motion in the joint. A physical therapist can teach various stretching or stabilizing exercises that can help reduce the pain. Options to stabilize the SI joint can include manual therapy, which can be very helpful. Sometimes, a sacroiliac belt, a device that wraps around the hips to help stabilize the SI joints, can also help the SI joint pain.

Injections into the SI joint can provide both diagnosis and treatment. The injections can be repeated up to three times a year. Injections work best when they are given using *fluoroscopy* (low-dose X-rays).

If other treatments fail and pain continues to interfere with normal activities, surgery might be an option. Surgery for SI dysfunction typically involves a fusion of the SI joints. In this surgery, the cartilage covering the surfaces of the SI joints is removed and the bones are held together with plates and screws until they grow together (*fuse*). This eliminates all motion at the SI joints. Surgery should only be considered if other less invasive treatments have not been successful.

CASE HISTORY

Richard was injured during a motor vehicle accident (MVA) and developed pain in his right sacroiliac joint. An X-ray-guided (*fluoroscopic*) injection of his right SI joint was done using a numbing medication (local anesthetic) and a small amount of steroid, which relieved his pain. This confirmed the SI joint as the source of pain.

He was then treated with manual therapy directed at treating the SI joint to help maintain neutral alignment of the sacroiliac joint. Like other forms of back pain, identifying the source of the pain before starting physical therapy is important in successfully designing a physical therapy program that works. Surgery for the SI joint is rare.

SECTION III

Treatment Options to Reduce Your Back Pain

CHAPTER 12

Five Tips to Reduce Back Pain With Physical Therapy

What good is physical therapy?

How does physical therapy help to reduce back pain?

Can I do the exercises at home?

How do exercises help when I have back pain?

These are typical questions I hear when I recommend physical therapy. I hope the tips below will be beneficial to you.

FIVE TIPS TO REDUCE BACK PAIN WITH PHYSICAL THERAPY

Patients with back pain often ask me, "How will physical therapy help me with my back pain?" and "If I am hurting, how will exercise help me?"

Not all physical therapy programs are suited for everyone. Therefore, patients should discuss their medical history with their qualified health care professionals before beginning treatment. However, a well-trained physical therapist can apply a variety of treatments, such as heat, ice, electrical stimulation, and muscle energy techniques to areas where back pain originates.

There are five areas where physical therapy can be highly beneficial in the treatment of low back pain:

1. Teaching proper body mechanics
2. Providing postural recommendations
3. Teaching specific exercises to increase flexibility and to strengthen abdominal and low back musculature
4. Improving weight control
5. Providing manual therapy techniques

If you believe that you don't have the time to participate in a physical therapy program, perhaps these benefits will change your mind.

1. UNDERSTANDING PROPER BODY MECHANICS

An understanding of proper body mechanics can reduce your need for medication and keep your spine healthy. An individualized physical therapy program can be helpful. Physical therapists help patients learn how to take care of their backs and how to manage recurrent episodes of back pain, thereby reducing the need for medications.

Body mechanics describes the way we move as we perform our daily activities. It focuses on how we sit, stand, bend, lift, and even how we sleep. Poor body mechanics can be the cause of back problems. When we don't move correctly, the spine is subjected to abnormal stresses that can lead to the degeneration of spinal structures like discs and joints and can result in unnecessary wear and tear over time. It is very important to understand proper body mechanics in order to keep your spine healthy.

2. PROVIDING POSTURAL RECOMMENDATIONS

In my extensive experience of treating patients with back pain, I have seen time and time again the importance of postural recommendations in relieving their pain. Good posture is key in the prevention and control of back pain, and who is better suited to teach patients about postural recommendations than the physical therapist?

While often overlooked, a good understanding of proper sitting and standing postures can greatly eliminate back pain. People often associate back pain with lifting, but poor posture is also a culprit. Although improper lifting can result in back pain, correcting your posture is key. The deleterious effects of improper sitting can result in significant pain.

It's easy to develop bad habits. However, good body mechanics are based on good posture.

Being aware of your posture during all of your daily activities is the best way to ensure you are using good body mechanics. Education on proper posture and body mechanics is an essential part in reducing and preventing back pain and thereby helping to avoid surgery.

3. TEACHING SPECIFIC EXERCISES

As your back pain improves, your physical therapist can teach you specific exercises to increase flexibility, to strengthen the back and abdominal muscles, and to improve your posture.

Stretching increases flexibility, and increased flexibility helps you comfortably and fluidly perform activities of daily living. The increased flexibility will also help reduce the risk of muscle, joint, and tendon injuries. Stretching also can often alleviate low back pain. Muscle tightness in the quadriceps, hamstrings, hip flexors, and low back muscles is a common cause of low back pain. Stretching these muscles will often eliminate the pain.

In physical therapy, strengthening the muscles of the abdomen, back, and legs helps to reduce the symptoms of nerve compression.

4. IMPROVING WEIGHT CONTROL

As you gain strength in your lower extremities, abdominal, and back muscles, your endurance will improve. This will give you more energy, which, in turn, can help you better control your weight and even lose weight when accompanied with the monitoring of your caloric intake. As your body tones and your stamina increases, you will improve your exercise tolerance and lose some body fat. Studies have shown that back pain decreases when you are at your ideal body weight.

5. PROVIDING MANUAL THERAPY TECHNIQUES

Physical therapists use a wide variety of manual techniques to help restore normal alignment and joint movement. A well-trained manual physical therapist can mobilize joints in a manner that a patient cannot do his or herself. They teach patients how to maintain good alignment once it is properly restored.

The exercises you learn in physical therapy can be done at home. By adhering to your postural recommendations, maintaining good body mechanics, and performing your home exercise program, you can control your back pain better.

By performing exercises for your back on a regular basis, you can help to prevent your back pain from recurring, correct current back problems, help prevent new ones, and relieve back pain, particularly after an injury. Proper exercise strengthens back muscles that support the spine and strengthens the abdomen, arms, and legs, reducing strain on the back. Exercise also strengthens bones and reduces the risk of falls and injuries.

IN SUMMARY

There are many different causes of back pain. Therefore, it is important that your physical therapy program be individualized to meet your specific needs. Working with your physician and physical therapist can help to reduce your back pain. An individualized physical therapy program where your physician works closely with your physical therapist can be beneficial to you in helping to control your back pain. For lasting benefits, it is important to continue to perform the exercises you learn in physical therapy at home on a routine basis once the physical therapy program has been discontinued. This way, you can continue to strengthen the muscles of your abdomen, arms, and legs and help to control your back pain.

Physical therapy is a key component of the treatment of spinal disorders. In some cases, physical therapy may be prescribed as your primary treatment. However, if you have had spinal surgery, at an appropriate time after surgery, your physician will prescribe a trial of physical therapy. Physical therapy can help patients to move forward in their recovery and return to their activities of daily living. This will be a critical component in your recovery following spinal surgery.

CHAPTER 13

Should You Use Ice or Heat?

This is a question I am asked often. Ice is usually preferred. However, there are those who say they can't tolerate the cold. I understand. Who would choose to take a cold bubble bath? No one. However, for acute back pain, *ice* works best; gel ice packs work the very best.

Remember these key points:

1. You can never go wrong with ice.
2. Always ice for the first 72 hours.
3. If you use heat and within a half hour to an hour you feel stiffer and more sore, then you should be icing.
4. Use moist heat, not dry heat.

5. Use a wet towel between the heat/ice and your skin. We need this protective layer.

ICE

I once sprained my back and I had spasms. If this has happened to you, you might have no idea whether you should use ice or heat. But ice is what you need. Ice is your best friend. You can't go wrong with ice. Ice generally will not harm you. Ice decreases the inflammatory process, which causes swelling. If there is less swelling, there will be less impairment after the inflammation has stopped. Ice also decreases the sensation of pain. If there is no pain, then the muscles that are in spasm and protecting the body are allowed to relax.

I recommend icing when there is:

1. Less than 72 hours after injury; for example, after a lumbar strain or sprain
2. A chronic injury that has recently become more aggravated; ice is *excellent* for spasms
3. Warmth and swelling of the area

When applying ice:

- For small areas, you can use an ice cube and massage it for seven minutes or until it is numb.

- For moderately sized areas, use an ice pack so it can wrap around the area. I recommend gel ice packs. These work well.

- Never apply the ice directly to the skin.

- A towel or pillow case should be placed between the body and the ice.

- Ice should be applied for 10 to 15 minutes, depending on the thickness of the area where it is being applied. The thicker the area, the more time is needed, but do not exceed 15 minutes. Icing should be performed every two hours. Use it several times.

- When icing, you should expect to first experience a feeling of cold followed by a burning sensation, then achy, and finally numbness.

Ice should not be used if you have:

1. Raynaud's disease
2. Rheumatoid arthritis
3. Cold hypersensitivity
4. Cold allergy
5. Diabetes with vascular disease
6. Peripheral vascular disease
7. Malignancy
8. Impaired sensation

9. Cryoglobulinemia
10. Paroxysmal cold hemoglobinuria
11. Fragile skin because you are elderly

HEAT

Heat should *never* be used immediately after an injury. I recommend heat when:

1. There are tight muscles.
2. The condition is chronic (over three months).
3. When the injury is no longer inflamed or warm to the touch.

Heat increases blood flow to an area, which brings all of the vital nutrients it needs for injury repair. In addition, it has a calming effect and relaxes muscles, thus allowing them to be more flexible, which, in turn, allows you to have increased mobility. Heat also helps reduce pain as well as muscle spasm.

I recommend using moist heat. This can be done by soaking the area in a hot bath or heating up a wet towel until it is comfortably hot. Moist heat penetrates deep beyond the skin.

Heating should be performed for 15 to 20 minutes. Check the skin every once in a while to make sure that it is not burning.

If someone tells you your back looks like a checkerboard, the heat was either too hot, or you kept it on your skin too long.

Heat should *not* be used if you have:

1. Malignancy
2. Impaired sensation (for example, from diabetes)
3. Infections
4. Impaired blood flow
5. Multiple sclerosis
6. Pregnancy
7. Deep vein thrombosis

For an injury that has occurred more than 36 hours earlier, we are not completely sure whether heat or cold is required. If you use heat and feel good immediately after using it, but then within a half hour or hour, you experience feeling more stiff and tight, this is likely an indication that there is still an inflammatory process occurring; therefore, you should use ice.

CHAPTER 14

Five Secrets to Reduce Back Pain While at Work

P atients always ask: How can I do my job when I have back pain? Are there exercises I can do at work to relieve my back pain? Let's examine the secrets below that will help you reduce your back pain at work.

1. **Strive to keep an ideal weight.** Obesity alone does not cause back pain; however, being overweight increases your risk of having back pain. Performing isometrics such as tightening the muscles of the buttocks and legs while sitting is an easy way to burn extra calories and maintain a healthy weight.

2. **Purchase a pedometer and walk 10,000 steps per day.** This will improve your cardiovascular status, help you lose weight, and therefore reduce your risk of low back pain. Park your car a little farther away from your office to increase your steps. Take the stairs instead of the elevator. Start taking those extra steps today, and you will see how easy it is to accomplish your goal.

3. **Take a postural break after sitting one to two hours.** Aim to never sit any longer than two hours continuously. Less is better, but this is sometimes difficult to achieve in the workplace. Get into the routine of walking to the bathroom or going to the break room to get a glass of water after two hours of continuous sitting. Your back muscles need a break. Sitting continuously is one of the worst things you can do to your back because it increases the risk of back pain.

4. **Improve your sitting posture.** Improving your posture is an essential step to reducing back pain. Place the lumbar roll in the small part of your back. Lumbar rolls can be purchased at many stores like Target or Wal-Mart or a sporting goods store.

   While at your desk, sit correctly with your shoulders relaxed, arms supported by an armrest, feet flat on the floor, and your knees level with your hips. Sitting correctly will help to improve your posture. Move the monitor and keyboards forward to a location that does not encourage slouching. Correct sitting posture will help reduce your risk of back pain.

5. **Perform extension exercises.** We spend a great deal of time flexing our backs when performing activities like brushing our teeth, putting on clothes, and getting files out of a cabinet. Therefore, we need to counteract these flexion activities with extension. Take the time to do some *extension exercises* while at work.

   Extension exercises can easily be done by standing with your hands on your hips and bending backward. Stand at your desk and do a set of 10 a couple of times throughout the day, or during your break, go to the restroom and do a set of 10. (However, if you have lumbar or spinal stenosis, you should avoid this stretching exercise.)

Remember, before beginning any exercise program, check with your physician first. Don't do any exercise that causes pain. These five secrets can help reduce your risk of back pain.

CHAPTER 15

Seven Secrets to Reduce Back Pain While Watching Television

WHAT CAN YOU DO AT HOME TO REDUCE YOUR BACK PAIN?

Americans watch television an average of four hours per day. Start using some of the time you spend watching television to reduce your back pain. Simply incorporate as much movement as possible during your television time. Although obesity itself does not cause back pain, being overweight increases your risk of back pain. Make the effort to maintain an ideal body weight to reduce your risk of back pain.

Try these seven secrets to reduce back pain while watching television:

1. **Shed those extra pounds while walking in place.** Walking is an excellent way to shed extra pounds and to improve your cardiovascular health as well.

    While watching television, walking in place for 30 minutes is an excellent activity to incorporate. If you find that walking in place during a television program causes you to lose track of the program, you can limit this activity to only when the commercials are aired. There are about 15 minutes of commercials during a one-hour program. If keeping track of your walking time doesn't work for you, purchase a pedometer and strive to walk 10,000 steps per day. Arrange to walk in place during your favorite television show, and see how easy it is to accumulate the steps. *Start stepping today!*

2. **After sitting and watching television for 30 minutes, take a postural break.** Never sit any longer than two hours continuously. Walk to the bathroom or go to the kitchen and get a glass of water after sitting 30 minutes. This will give your back muscles a much needed break. Prolonged sitting is one of the worst things you

can do to your back because this alone increases the risk of back pain.

3. **Place a lumbar roll in your chair.** This will improve your sitting posture and reduce your back pain.

4. **Use stability balls to improve your posture.** Stability balls are great for the back. Simply sitting on a stability ball will help to improve your posture. Correctly sitting on a stability ball will help increase your abdominal strength. You can find these large balls at many stores. Purchase one and start increasing the strength of your back muscles today.

5. **Increase the strength of your core with a stability ball.** This can easily be done while watching television. Use the stability ball to perform simple exercises like wall slides that can easily be done during commercials.

6. **For advanced strengthening of your core, try this one.** While on all fours, tighten your stomach and raise either your right or left leg and the opposite arm. Keep your back rigid. Repeat 10 times per set. Do two sets per day.

7. **Perform some extension exercises.** We spend a great amount of time flexing our backs; therefore, we need to perform extension exercises to counteract these activities. These exercises can easily be done while standing

and placing your hands on your hips and bending backward. (However, if you have spinal stenosis, avoid this stretching exercise.)

Before beginning any exercise program, always check with your physician. Never do any exercise that causes pain.

Get started today, using these seven secrets to reduce your back pain.

CHAPTER 16

Twelve Common Tips to Prevent Back Pain

Too often, back pain destroys vacations and holidays. How do I handle cooking for the holidays? What can I do to reduce my pain when putting up decorations? Shopping kills me, what can I do?

The 12 tips and illustrations on the following pages will help you deal with some of these questions about how to handle and remove back pain from your vacations and holidays.

TWELVE COMMON TIPS TO PREVENT BACK PAIN

1. Have you ever wondered if your weight has any effect on your back pain? While certainly all overweight people do not have back pain, extra weight can increase the risk of low back pain. Therefore, it is easy to walk four to five days per week for 30 to 60 minutes to help keep an ideal body weight and reduce your risk of back pain. So, why not take the time to shed those extra pounds by starting a walking program and reducing your risk of back pain? (See Figure 1.)

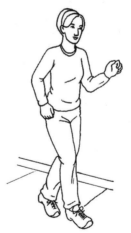

Figure 1. *Walking 30 to 60 minutes a day for four to five days per week will reduce your risk of back pain.*

2. Years ago in Michigan, I met a guy named Bill. Bill was a machinist who had degenerative disc disease. He always complained of an aching back. His pain usually did not radiate to his legs, but he had problems with sitting and with moving. He described his pain as a throbbing, aching pain that sometimes was horrible.

Living in Michigan, one of the things that Bill had to learn how to do was shovel snow. He told me that every winter, he had a lot of back pain. After talking to Bill for a long period of time and after getting to know him, I learned that his back pain was usually exacerbated after the first snowfall. When I saw Bill, he would come in all slumped over to the point where it was even difficult for him to stand. Bill finally learned how to shovel snow without exacerbating his pain.

Figure 2 illustrates what I recommended for Bill, that he needed to be careful when shoveling snow. I told him he should stand with his knees bent and push from the end of the handle to relieve pressure on his back and avoid twisting his back. This

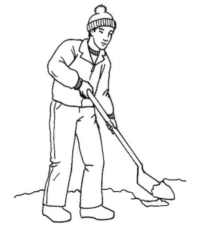

Figure 2. *The correct way to shovel snow to avoid putting pressure on your back.*

simple maneuver made a major difference in Bill's life by reducing his risk of back pain.

3. Over the years, I have noticed a lot of patients come to me complaining of back pain right around the time when they do their spring cleaning. I have observed that there are patients whom I see every year around March. They are cleaning out their closets and cleaning their home and getting ready for the spring.

Have you ever noticed that after vacuuming, your back pain becomes worse? If this is the case, take the advice that I gave Paul, a 60-year-old gentleman who always helped his wife with spring cleaning. I told Paul that he had to learn to be safe with spring cleaning. When doing household chores like vacuuming, I recommend that you put all of your weight on the back foot, then step forward with the other foot as you push the vacuum

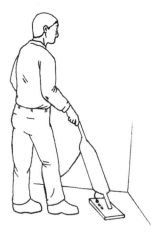

Figure 3. *The correct way to vacuum to avoid back pain.*

cleaner forward and back. Use the back foot as a pivot when turning and when performing your household chores; take my advice and avoid twisting your back. Figure 3 illustrates the advice I gave Paul.

4. In April, I see a lot of accountants and bookkeepers, and I started wondering why. Over the years, I have found that the long hours they spend sitting at their desks and computers during tax season can exacerbate their back pain.

I say, do not let Uncle Sam cause you back pain! When doing your taxes, remember: sitting puts a lot of stress on the lower back. You need to do what your mother recommended: sit up straight, keep your shoulders relaxed, feet flat on the floor, and your knees level with your hips. (See Figure 4.)

It is also important to take a break and get up every one to

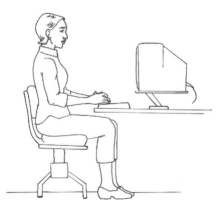

Figure 4. *Sitting puts a lot of stress on your lower back. Sitting correctly will prevent back pain.*

two hours for a quick stretch. Remember: prolonged sitting is one of the most common causes of back pain. Prolonged sitting may cause the muscles that support the spine to tighten and cause pain. So, do not be like the accountants and bookkeepers who are working on taxes in the wee hours during the month of April—take a stretch break and protect your back.

5. Many people enjoy gardening because it is so relaxing. As a child and young adult, I always enjoyed having a vegetable garden. Watching flowers bloom and harvesting vegetables brings joy to many people. This is a relaxing time when one can clear the mind and enjoy this traditional American pastime. When it is time to do your gardening, enjoy it. Do not let the gardening and lawn chores get the best of you. When weeding or planting, do what I have recommended over the years: kneel

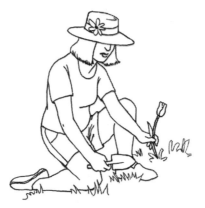

Figure 5. Enjoy your gardening, but remember to bend at the hips to avoid back pain. You can also use a stool while gardening to prevent back pain.

or squat; do not bend at the waist. Bending at the waist only increases your back pain. (See Figure 5.)

6. When summer comes, we all love to travel. However, going on long trips can certainly increase back pain. Why? Because we find ourselves in cars driving long distances and doing what I said we should avoid—prolonged sitting. If you are going to drive, make sure that you take a postural break every couple of hours, get out of the car, and stretch. Otherwise, you are going to put extra stress on your back, and by the time you reach your destination, you might have back pain.

When you travel, leave the back pain at home. Remember to balance the load; that is, when carrying your bags, put one bag in one hand and one in the other. It's also a good idea to alternate occasionally. Figure 6 demonstrates the proper way to carry

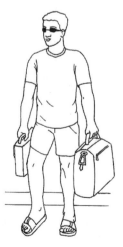

Figure 6. *Balance the load!*

your bags. This is what I have recommended to my patients over the years so that they can enjoy their travel time without back pain. Some of them, however, will insist on putting all their bags on one side—one on the shoulder and one in their hand—and this is the reason that I see them every summer. So, take my advice and balance the load. This will help you to reduce the risk of back pain and have a better chance of enjoying your vacation.

Ladies, it is important to limit what we put in our purses as well. Too often, I see women with purses weighing more than seven pounds! That's the weight of a newborn! I recommend they reduce the weight in their purses and carry their purses in one hand and their briefcases in the other hand.

7. When school is out, have fun with your child and do not let childcare activities cause you back pain. Remember: bend

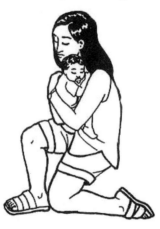

Figure 7. *This is the safe way to lift your child to avoid back pain.*

with your knees. Do not pick up your child with outstretched arms. Bring the baby or child close to your chest before lifting. Using this simple technique will help you avoid back pain. Take a look at Figure 7, which illustrates the safe way to lift your child and avoid back pain.

8. Four out of five adults will experience back pain at some point in their lives. However, if you are going to the beach, lift the coolers using your legs. Stand close to the cooler with your feet shoulder-width apart. Put one foot slightly in front of the other. Pick up the cooler and bring it close to your body. Remember: never pick up a cooler or a box with outstretched arms. If you do so, you are increasing the risk of having back pain. Instead, lift using your legs, and this will help you avoid back pain and enjoy the beach this year.

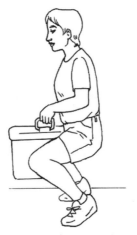

Figure 8. *The correct way to pick up a cooler and avoid back pain.*

9. Ladies, let's stay pain-free. When you are purchasing shoes for the fall, remember: high heels may be stylish, but they often cause back pain. Choose styles with no more than two-inch heels with a wide heel base. (See my article in the June 2003 issue of *Redbook*. This is what I told *Redbook*, and this is what I am telling you.) While this type of shoe may not win a fashion award, it will certainly help to reduce your risk of back pain. Take a look at the shoes in Figure 9 and remember: the higher the heel, the more likely you are to have back pain.

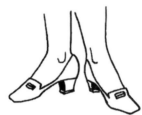

Figure 9. *Remember: the higher the heel, the more likely you are to have back pain.*

10. Fall is a special time of year, and I love watching the leaves as they change colors. When leaves fall, someone has to gather them. Yes, it is okay to rake the leaves, but do it safely. Avoid pushing with your back, and stand with your feet shoulder-width apart, one foot in front of the other. Try to keep your back straight, and do not bend at the waist. These simple techniques will help you to reduce your risk of back pain when you have to rake the leaves. (See Figure 10.)

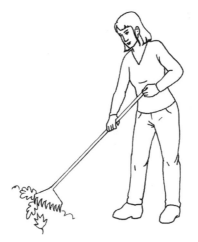

Figure 10. *It is okay to rake the leaves, but do it safely.*

11. There are patients whom I see every year around Thanksgiving, and I used to think that they just liked to come in and wish me a Happy Thanksgiving. I have been seeing them for many years. I finally figured out why I see them every year in November with an exacerbated case of back pain.

Thanksgiving is a special family time where we all get together and enjoy family gatherings. But with family gatherings, you know there is usually is a big meal, and with a big meal, well, what is that one thing that we all hate to do after we have a big meal?

Sweet potato pie, dressing, turkey, potato salad, bean casserole, mama's special rolls; they all taste good, but at the end of the dinner, somebody has to do the dishes. After Thanksgiving dinner, yes, the dishes must be done, but this should not cause back pain.

If you're the lucky one who is washing the dishes, put one foot on a stool or on the ledge of the sink cabinet. Avoid leaning. These simple techniques will help you finish the Thanksgiving dinner without exacerbating back pain or preventing it from occurring in the first place. Not only will you be thankful for your wonderful friends and family and the fabulous dinner you just enjoyed, but you will also be thankful that you followed my advice and put one foot on a stool when you washed your dishes this year and reduced your risk of back pain after Thanksgiving dinner. (See Figure 11.)

12. Holiday seasons can be filled with a lot of special times for all of us, and we are much too busy to be worried about back

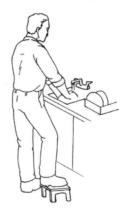

Figure 11. To avoid back pain when washing dishes, place one foot on a stool.

pain. When you are doing your holiday shopping, remember what I said earlier: balance the load, put one bag in one hand, and one in the other. Do not try to carry all of your bags in one arm. Remember to alternate occasionally.

I want you to enjoy the holidays, so be careful when getting decorations out of the closet. Use that stool that you used when you were washing the dishes to reach items that are above shoulder level. Do not stand on your toes trying to reach items that are out of reach; stand on the stool to reach them. You will find that this simple maneuver will help to reduce your risk of back pain and allow you to have pleasant holidays. (See Figure 12.)

Remember these 12 tips; if integrated into your daily life, they can help prevent low back pain.

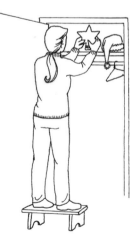

Figure 12. *Use a stool to reach objects out of reach in a closet instead of stretching for them.*

SECTION IV

When Is a Doctor Needed?

CHAPTER 17

When Should You
See a Doctor?

A fter an acute (recent) event, if your back pain is severe or doesn't improve after three days, call your doctor. You should also get medical attention if you experience back pain following an injury. You should see your doctor if you have any of the following symptoms. These symptoms could be a sign of a serious problem that requires immediate treatment.

- Loss of bladder control
- Loss of bowel control
- Fever
- Pain after a fall or an injury

- Pain that becomes worse after rest
- Pain that wakes you up at night
- Severe back pain that doesn't improve with medication and relative rest
- Significant back pain that lasts for more than three days
- Trouble urinating
- Weakness, pain, or numbness in your legs
- Weight loss (unintentional)

Most people experiencing back pain recover quickly without loss of spinal function. However, if you do not have significant reduction in pain and inflammation after 72 hours of self-care, you should contact a doctor to diagnose the cause of your back pain.

REMEMBER THESE RED FLAGS

In rare cases, back pain can be a symptom of a serious problem such as a heart attack, cancer, pneumonia, a blood clot in the lung, or peptic ulcer disease.

To rule out more serious conditions, you should see a doctor immediately if you experience fever, drastic weight loss, weakness of the legs, back pain at rest, pain that keeps you awake, or loss of bladder or bowel control.

CHAPTER 18

Will You Need Surgery for Your Back Pain?

Choose Your Surgeon Wisely

Most low back pain can be treated without surgery. In fact, surgery is seldom required to treat back pain. The first line of treatment for low back pain is usually relative rest (a couple of days), physical therapy, and medication, followed by interventional techniques like epidural injections. Only 5% of patients will need spinal surgery, yet we tend to think of back surgery as the "Big Fix." Surgery is often looked upon as the treatment that will work if other approaches are not successful. This leads patients, sometimes out of desperation, to jump over the less invasive procedures and go right to the knife.

The decision to undergo back surgery should never be taken lightly. Back surgery is a last resort and should only be considered when nonsurgical treatment options have failed.

The only absolute indications for back surgery are:

- Progressive neurologic loss (legs are getting weaker)
- Loss of control of your bowel or bladder (this does not mean constipation)
- Prolonged incapacitating pain that is not relieved by nonsurgical treatments

If you need surgery, take time to find a qualified spine surgeon. Make sure you understand the goals of the surgery. Always ask your surgeon what the success rate is with the type of surgery he or she recommends for you. These statistics can help predict your surgical outcome and help you determine if surgery is your best choice.

Communication with your surgeon is important. Take time and choose a surgeon whom you relate well to. If you can't talk to the surgeon before the surgery, you won't suddenly be able to communicate better after your surgery.

Always get a second opinion before you undergo surgery.

Unless surgery is absolutely indicated, get a second opinion from a nonsurgical spine specialist (physical medicine and rehabilitation specialist, neurologist, or rheumatologist, etc.). If you tell a surgeon that exercise and other nonsurgical options did not help, that could tilt the decision toward an operation. Often, patients have not given other nonsurgical strategies a thorough trial. This is advice that a nonsurgical spine specialist will be able to provide.

After most surgeries for back pain, patients need to go to physical therapy to learn postural recommendations and how to adhere to good body mechanics (how to sit, how to lift correctly, etc.) and how to strengthen their core muscles to protect the spine. (See chapter 12 on physical therapy and body mechanics.)

WHAT ARE THE RISKS OF SURGERY?

Surgical risks include infection, bleeding, dural leak, nerve root damage, and all the possible general anesthetic risks (e.g., blood clots, pulmonary emboli, pneumonia, heart attack, or stroke). Most of these complications are rare, but increased risks are seen in certain situations: Conditions that increase the risk of surgery include smoking (or any nicotine intake); obesity; multilevel fusions; osteoporosis (thinning of the bones); diabetes; rheumatoid arthritis; or prior failed back surgery.

WILL THE SURGICAL PROCEDURE
TAKE AWAY YOUR PAIN?

Having surgery does not guarantee pain relief. Preventing back pain is key. Mother knows best; prevention is the best medicine. Doing what your mother taught you about sitting up straight and not slouching is good medicine to prevent and relieve back pain. If your nerves were severely damaged before surgery, you may experience some pain or numbness after surgery. Sometimes after surgery, you may have no improvement at all. Several years after surgery, sometimes your symptoms can reappear.

WILL YOU BE ABLE TO RETURN TO
YOUR JOB AFTER SURGERY?

This question is particularly important to have answered when a lumbar fusion is recommended. Too often, patients who are required to perform heavy lifting undergo a fusion without clearly understanding that the likelihood of returning to their jobs is very slim.

I want to empower you to take control of your back pain and realize that undergoing the surgeon's knife does not keep you from having back pain for life. It is through correctly learning how to perform your normal activities of daily living that will help you prevent **back** pain. This is why it is so important to learn the 12 steps to prevent back pain in chapter 16.

CHAPTER 19

What Is Pain Management?

People often erroneously think of treatment by a pain management specialist as consisting of only narcotic "painkillers." However, the practice of pain medicine or pain management is "diagnosis driven," just like other medical specialties. Just as one goes to a cardiologist for an evaluation of heart disease and receives treatment based on a unique diagnosis, a visit to a pain management specialist results in unique treatment because every patient with pain is also different. The discipline of pain medicine is concerned with the prevention, evaluation, diagnosis, treatment, and rehabilitation of painful disorders.

Pain affects more Americans than diabetes, heart disease, and cancer combined. There are approximately 116 million Americans with chronic pain, defined as "pain that has lasted more than three months," and 25 million people with acute pain. Acute pain begins suddenly and is usually sharp in quality. It serves as a warning of disease or a threat to the body. Acute pain might be mild and last just a moment, or it might be severe and last for weeks or months. Usually, in most cases, acute pain does not last longer than three months. It disappears when the underlying cause of pain has been treated or has healed. Unrelieved acute pain, however, might lead to chronic pain.

Like other doctors, the pain management specialist must examine each patient and create a treatment plan based on the patient's symptoms, examination, and other findings. For example, the cardiologist must first examine you and make several determinations. These include deciding whether your heart disease will respond to weight loss and exercise; whether you have high blood pressure and need medication to lower your blood pressure; whether your cholesterol is elevated and you need medication to lower your cholesterol; whether you have a blockage and need an interventional procedure; or, as a last resort, whether you might need to be referred to a cardiac surgeon for coronary artery bypass surgery.

Not all patients with heart disease take the same medications.

It depends upon the cause of the problem. Just as there are different treatment options available for heart disease, there are a vast number of treatment options available for spinal (back) pain.

While patients may go to a pain management physician because they "hurt," just as they go to a cardiologist because they have heart problems, all pain does not respond to narcotics. It is an unfortunate and common misconception that if patients go to a pain management doctor they will be treated with narcotics. Treatments for spinal (back) pain vary just like treatments for heart disease vary. It depends on what the cause is.

First of all, it is important to understand that there are different types of spinal (back) pain. One might have muscular pain, ligamentous pain, joint pain, bone pain, pain due to a herniated disc, pain from a fracture, or pain from a pinched nerve or a nerve injury. Pain medicines are prescribed based upon the source and cause of the pain.

Some patients who go to a pain management doctor never take pain medications. They may respond to an injection, other interventions, bracing, or to physical therapy. Our knowledge has increased to where we understand more on how poor posture and walking improperly all perpetuate musculoskeletal pain. With the sophisticated use of exercises tailored to a patient's specific needs, physical therapy may be very helpful and solve the problem by itself.

An evaluation by a physical therapist may reveal that the patient's pain is a result of poor movement, tight or stiff muscles, weak musculature, or postural problems. For example, we know that patients who have degenerative disc disease—where the disc between two bones has started to wear and tear—can decrease the pressure on the disc by performing exercises to increase their core musculature and eliminate or reduce their back pain.

Like the cardiologist who performs interventional procedures such as cardiac catheterizations, pain management physicians perform interventional procedures to eliminate or reduce pain, and surgery, as in other areas of medicine, should always be the last resort.

When you initially go to your cardiologist because of a minor problem, I am sure that most of you would not ask, "Do I need surgery?" One usually wants to explore other options before surgical interventions are explored. From experience, I have learned that patients do best with treatment by a pain management specialist when they come with the same open mind and attitude where they are willing to explore numerous options and not become focused primarily on getting narcotics or thinking that surgery is their only option. I used the example of the cardiologist because I know that most of us would prefer that the cardiologist explore all options before referring us to a cardiac surgeon. This is the same approach that patients should use when they have orthopedic or spinal problems. Always ask about nonsurgical options for your orthopedic or spinal pain.

The pain management physician, like the cardiologist, does not perform surgery. The cardiologist does interventional techniques, prescribes medications, and oversees your cardiac rehab program. Likewise, a pain management physician manages and directs your physical therapy or rehabilitation program, prescribes medications, and performs interventional procedures. Both the cardiologist and pain specialist will refer you to a surgeon when needed.

Timing is key to the success of your treatment. As you should not delay an evaluation for heart disease, neither should you continue to ignore spinal or orthopedic pain and wait too long before seeking an evaluation with a pain specialist. I have seen far too many patients wait too late in their treatment before seeking care with a pain specialist. Like other specialties, early intervention might lead to a better outcome.

Pain management is a process. It consists of many treatment options, and more importantly, the treatment for your pain may not be the same as it is for your neighbor's; just like a pacemaker may be the treatment of choice for your spouse but not the treatment of choice for you when you see a cardiologist.

IN SUMMARY

With advances in pain management, there are a number of treatment options, and narcotics are not the treatment of choice for everyone who sees a pain management specialist.

Never allow a pain management specialist to perform a procedure if he or she has not performed a neuromuscular examination on you before the procedure.

A neuromuscular examination is important in determining what the best procedure is for you.

A physician board certified in pain medicine can have training in various specialties, such as physical medicine and rehabilitation (physiatrist); neurology/psychiatry; family medicine; radiology; emergency medicine; or anesthesiology. Not all of them perform procedures, and not all of them will prescribe pain medications. You need to take the time to choose the best pain management specialist who fits your needs.

If you need procedures and medications, you should look for a physician who does both.

Most pain specialists treat acute pain. Therefore, you should see them before you see a surgeon, since only 5% of patients will need back surgery.

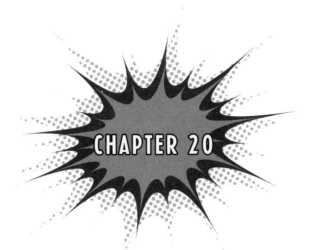

Myths About Back Pain

ike everything else, there are myths about back pain. I will discuss a few of them in hopes that you will not be alarmed when you hear them.

MYTH: DON'T LIFT HEAVY OBJECTS

It's not necessarily how much you lift; it's how you lift. Of course, you shouldn't lift anything that might be too heavy for you. When you lift, squat close to the object with your back straight and head up. Stand, using your legs to lift the load. Do not twist or bend your body while lifting or you may hurt your back. Bring the object close to your chest before lifting.

MYTH: BED REST IS THE BEST CURE

Yes, resting can help an acute injury or strain/sprain that causes back pain. But it's a myth that you should stay in bed. Studies show that people who rest less and try to stay active feel better faster. Try to rest for no longer than 24 to 48 hours. Resting longer can make your back pain worse.

FACT: MORE POUNDS, MORE PAIN

Staying fit helps prevent back pain. Back pain is most common among people who are out of shape. And obesity stresses the back.

MYTH: SKINNY MEANS PAIN-FREE

Anyone can get back pain. In fact, people who are too thin, such as those suffering from anorexia, an eating disorder, may suffer bone loss resulting in fractured or crushed vertebrae.

MYTH: EXERCISE IS BAD FOR BACK PAIN

Regular exercise prevents back pain. For people suffering an acute injury resulting in lower back pain, an exercise program that begins with gentle exercises should be started and gradually increased in intensity. Once the acute pain subsides, an exercise regimen may help prevent a future recurrence of back pain. Treatment by a physical therapist can be helpful.

MYTH: FIRMER MATTRESSES ARE BETTER

Depending on your sleep habits and the cause of your back pain, different people may need different mattresses. However, I recommend that you avoid water beds since they offer limited support. Memory foam mattresses can be utilized in cases where a patient has a very rigid spine.

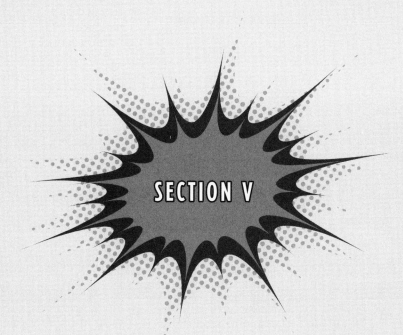

SECTION V

Action Steps You Must Take

CHAPTER 21

Keep a Pain Diary

WHY KEEP A PAIN DIARY?

f you have chronic back pain—pain that has lasted more than three months—keep a pain diary to help facilitate communication with your doctor.

You should keep a log of your pain: when, where, and how much your back hurts; what activities you did during the day; and anything else you think might be important.

Keeping a pain diary may help you and your doctor better understand your pain and determine connections that you might have otherwise missed.

Discussing things that increased your pain, for example, if it feels more intense when you sit too long at work, can be helpful in treating your pain.

The diary can also help you track which medical treatments and lifestyle changes work best for you.

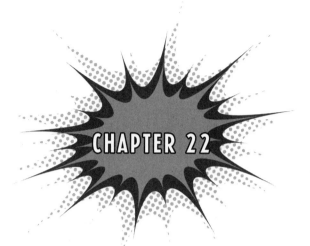

Pay Attention to Your Health Each Month

A s the year goes by, pay attention to the designated Health Awareness Months to ensure that you have taken care of your preventive tests throughout the year. These are important months for your health.

JANUARY IS GLAUCOMA AWARENESS MONTH

Words to live by:

> *"There is a great deal of pain in life and perhaps the only pain that can be avoided is the pain that comes from trying to avoid pain."* -R.D. Laing

Glaucoma is one of the leading causes of blindness in the United States, and the most common cause of blindness in African Americans. More than three million people in the United States have glaucoma, but half do not realize it because there are often no warning symptoms.

FEBRUARY IS AMERICAN HEART MONTH

Words to live by:

> *"With every new answer unfolded, Science has consistently discovered at least three new questions." -Wernher Von Braun*

Love yourself this month, and treat yourself to a total body massage to reduce muscle tension. Stress can lead to tight, painful muscles and amplify back pain. Also, the risks of heart disease and stroke increase with age. Of American women aged 18 to 64, 19.5% smoke, putting them at increased risk for a heart attack or stroke.

MARCH IS COLORECTAL CANCER AWARENESS MONTH

Words to live by:

> *"How poor are they who have not patience! What wound did ever heal, but by degrees?" -William Shakespeare*

Colorectal cancer is the second leading cause of cancer death after lung cancer in the United States.

APRIL IS ALCOHOL AWARENESS MONTH

Words to live by:

> *"Sometimes our light goes out but is blown into a flame by another human being. Each of us owes deepest thanks to those who have rekindled this light."*
> *-Albert Schweitzer*

Research has long shown that the abuse of alcohol, tobacco, and illicit drugs is the single most serious health problem in the United States, straining the health care system, burdening the economy, and contributing to the health problems and death of millions of Americans every year. Today, substance abuse causes more deaths, illnesses, and disabilities than any other preventable health condition.

MAY IS NATIONAL ARTHRITIS MONTH

Words to live by:

> *"Doubt is a pain too lonely to know that faith is his twin brother." -Kahlil Gibran*

Arthritis is the nation's leading cause of disability among Americans over age 15.

Arthritis limits everyday activities such as walking, dressing, and bathing for more than seven million Americans.

JUNE IS NATIONAL SAFETY MONTH

Words to live by:

> *"What lies behind us and what lies before us*
> *are tiny matters compared to what lies with us."*
> *-Ralph Waldo Emerson*

More people are injured in their homes than anywhere else.

Never give prescription medication to anyone other than the person to whom it was prescribed.

JULY IS EYE INJURY PREVENTION MONTH

Words to live by:

> *"How far you go in life depends on your being ten-*
> *der with the young, compassionate with the aged, sym-*
> *pathetic with the striving, and tolerant of the weak*
> *and strong. Because someday in your life you will have*
> *been all of these." -George Washington Carver*

More than one million people suffer from eye injuries each year in the United States, and 90% of them could have been prevented with appropriate protective eyewear.

AUGUST IS NATIONAL IMMUNIZATION AWARENESS MONTH

Words to live by:

> *"Wisdom doesn't automatically come with old age. Nothing does—except wrinkles. It's true some wines improve with age. But only if the grapes were good in the first place." -Abigail Van Buren*

In the United States, approximately 48,000 adults die each year from vaccine-preventable diseases.

SEPTEMBER IS PROSTATE CANCER AWARENESS MONTH

Words to live by:

> *"Forget Injuries, never forget kindnesses." -Confucius*

Prostate cancer is the most commonly diagnosed cancer in America among men. All men of appropriate age should ask their doctors to be screened for prostate cancer. Starting at age 50, men should talk to their doctor about testing. If you are African American or have a father or brother who had prostate cancer before age 65, talk to your doctor about testing at age 45. This talk should occur at age 40 for men with two or more close relatives with prostate cancer before age 65.

OCTOBER IS NATIONAL BREAST CANCER AWARENESS MONTH

Words to live by:

> *"The best way to cheer yourself up is to try to cheer somebody else up." –Mark Twain*

Breast cancer is the second-most common kind of cancer in women. About 1 in 8 (12%) women in the United States will develop invasive breast cancer during their lifetimes.

NOVEMBER IS AMERICAN DIABETES MONTH

Words to live by:

> *"Never stand begging for that which you have the power to earn." –Miguel de Cervantes*

About 29 million people in the United States have diabetes, while 1 out of 4 are unfortunately unaware that they have the disease.

DECEMBER IS NATIONAL DRUNK AND DRUGGED DRIVING PREVENTION MONTH

Words to live by:

"No one needs a smile as much as a person who fails to give one." –Author Unknown

In 2012, 10,322 people were killed in alcohol-impaired driving crashes, accounting for nearly one-third (31%) of all traffic-related deaths in the United States. Each year, approximately 16,000 people are killed in alcohol-related car crashes.

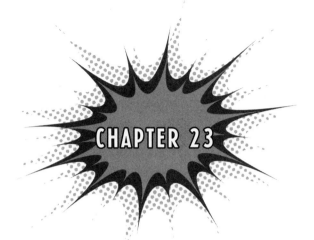

CHAPTER 23

Medical Logs

COMMIT TO BETTER HEALTH

This year, make a commitment to better health. Make your appointments now to see your doctors. Keep track of these important appointments on your Health Log.

Know your medications; keep a log of them, too. Too often, medication errors occur because patients don't know their medications. Don't let this happen to you.

Keep track of your injections. You need to know how many steroid injections you have had during the year.

Keep track of your surgeries so you can discuss what procedures you have undergone. This will also help to facilitate getting your records when needed.

Use the logs on the next pages to help you keep track of your health appointments, medications, injections, and surgeries.

IMPORTANT HEALTH APPOINTMENTS

EVALUATIONS	DATES
Back Evaluation	
Colonoscopy	
Dental Exam	
Eye Evaluation	
Mammogram/Pap Smear	
Orthopedic Evaluation	
Pain-Medicine Follow-Up	
Prostate Evaluation	
Routine Physical	

MEDICATION LIST

(include prescription drugs, over-the-counter medicines, and vitamins and supplements)

1. _____
2. _____
3. _____
4. _____
5. _____
6. _____
7. _____
8. _____
9. _____
10. _____
11. _____
12. _____
13. _____
14. _____
15. _____
16. _____
17. _____
18. _____
19. _____
20. _____

PROCEDURE LOG (INJECTIONS)

Dates	Site of injection	Doctor that performed injection

SURGERY LOG

Dates	Site of Surgery	Surgery Performed by

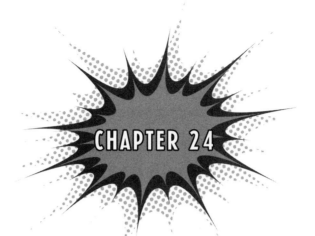

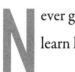

Help the Doctor to Help You

Never go to the doctor and say, "It just hurts." You need to learn how to tell your doctor where it hurts.

NINE STEPS TO A MORE EFFECTIVE VISIT WITH YOUR DOCTOR

These nine steps should help make your next visit with your doctor more effective and efficient. Health care is undergoing major changes, and doctors are challenged to see more patients and to complete more paperwork in the same amount of time. Therefore, patients today must be armed with information when they arrive for their doctors' visits. By bringing this nine-point checklist with completed information to your next doctor's visit, you will ensure that your time with your doctor was well spent. A little preparation will save you from wasting time and allow your doctor to spend more time focusing on you. It will also enhance the communication between you and your doctor. Take my advice and don't leave home without your checklist and these nine items:

1. Your insurance card and a photo ID. Inform the staff of changes in address and phone numbers. All patients need to understand their insurance coverage. Everyone needs to know their deductibles and copays. A lot of time is spent gathering this information, so be sure to provide accurate information to reduce your waiting time in the doctor's office.

2. Names, phone numbers, and dates of treatment by other health care providers or health care facilities (i.e., urgent care centers or emergency rooms) where you have been treated since your last visit. Gathering medical information can be a time-consuming process; the more accurate information you provide, the less time you will spend in this information-gathering process.

3. List of tests done since your last visit, including the name of the facilities where the testing occurred, and the

dates of the tests. Bring test results with you to your appointment. This will greatly reduce the time you will spend waiting on test results.

4. List of all current medications (include prescription drugs, over-the-counter medicines, and vitamins and supplements). Be sure to list the name of each medicine, dosage, and number of times you take the medicine each day. Include any allergies to medications, foods, or other products.

5. List describing any side effects of newly prescribed medications. This can include things like nausea, dizziness, constipation, and so on.

6. Statement describing your primary problem. Before you leave home, write one sentence describing the primary reason you want to be seen. In your own words, describe the symptoms of the main problem you want evaluated during your appointment. This will help with your discussion with your doctor.

You need to clearly describe the problems you are experiencing. Ask yourself: When did my problem start? How often does it occur? What makes it better or worse? If your problem causes pain, describe the pain. For example, merely saying, "My back hurts," does not give the doctor enough information to determine your diagnosis. Be specific to better assist your doctor in taking care of your needs. Doctors want to help you; however, you need to provide specific information to assist the doctor in the process.

7. Tell the receptionist about multiple problems. If you have several problems, you need to make sure you express this clearly when your appointment is initially made with the receptionist. This will allow the staff to schedule a longer appointment for your visit. Otherwise, if you make an appointment for one problem and you want to discuss several problems, the office might ask that you arrange a follow-up for additional concerns.

When you want to discuss multiple problems, it is *extremely* important that you bring a written statement describing each problem—discussing the symptoms as indicated in point number 6—so you can discuss this information with your doctor. This will greatly help the doctor and the staff in taking care of you.

8. A concise list of questions. Think about the questions you have for the doctor before you leave home. Ask your questions while the doctor is in the examination room with you. Once the doctor has started examining another patient, it is difficult for the doctor to return to your examination room. Creating your question list before you leave home should increase the likelihood that you receive answers to your concerns in a timely manner. General or routine questions can be answered by staff while waiting on the doctor.

9. Pen and paper. This will allow you to make a note of any advice or information that your doctor gives you. Write down your diagnosis; this will allow you to read about your condition on your doctor's website.

Be sure to bring your nine-item checklist to your next doctor's visit. Each time you return for follow-up visits, continue to update your checklist to ensure that you make the most out of your doctor's visit. Bring your checklist to all your doctors' visits.

Your good health is the mutual goal of the patient and the physician. Remember: preparation before your office visit can save you time in the doctor's office and lead to a more effective and efficient visit with your physician. Take my advice: don't leave home without your nine-point doctor visit checklist.

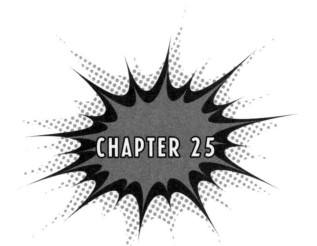

CHAPTER 25

Frequently Asked Questions About Back Pain

1. WHEN SHOULD I SEE A PAIN SPECIALIST?

I believe that too many patients seek care by a pain management specialist too late in the treatment process. Often, they come to me after they have undergone surgery, when, in fact, it is better to seek nonsurgical solutions first. Only 5% of patients will need back surgery.

Because pain and function are intimately related, many of my patients finally seek my expertise when they are no longer able to perform their activities of daily living. By this time, often their pain has become excruciating or unbearable. Due to their overwhelming pain, sometimes patients finally decide to seek pain management when they are no longer able to work, and their employer has asked that they have a functional assessment to determine their work capacity.

Physicians who are board certified in pain can have training in various specialties. However, before your doctor performs any interventional procedures, make sure he or she performs a neuromuscular examination.

Seek pain management early, preferably before surgery.

2. WHAT IS APPROPRIATE PAIN MANAGEMENT?

My primary goal in treating any patient with pain is to have a positive impact on improving the person's quality of life. While it is always my goal to alleviate a patient's pain, I explain to my patients that sometimes a pain-free state is not realistic. More importantly, I stress that the ultimate goal of appropriate pain management is to improve a patients' quality of life so that they can engage in their normal activities of daily living. Restoration of their functions should be given as much attention as reducing their pain.

If the patient has not responded to conservative treatment after six weeks, I recommend that the primary care physician refer the patient to a spine specialist, such as a physical medicine and rehabilitation specialist (physiatrist), a neurologist, neuro-surgeon, or orthopedic spine surgeon for further evaluation.

3. ARE THERE ANY PRECAUTIONS YOU TAKE PRIOR TO PRESCRIBING PAIN MEDICATIONS?

There are well-established guidelines to follow when one pre-scribes an opioid (narcotic) analgesic on a long-term basis. The patient must be willing to comply with six things:

1. Submit to periodic urine or blood drug screens
2. Consent and follow an Opioid Agreement
3. Designate one doctor to write the pain medications
4. Use one pharmacy for pain medications
5. Be compliant and take the medications as prescribed
6. Keep all follow-up appointments

Education about the use of opioid analgesics is important so the patient can understand that there are anticipated side effects, risks, and benefits.

4.   WHAT YOU CAN DO TO PREVENT BACK PAIN?

About 80% of us will experience back pain by age 55. Back pain is the second most common cause of disability for patients less than 45 years of age. Yet, by practicing good biomechanics, many of us can prevent back pain. I stress that it is important to incorporate these simple tips to prevent back pain:

1. When lifting an object, bend at the knees, straighten your back, and tighten your abdominals and buttocks.
2. When lifting objects, bring them close to the chest and do not lift any object with outstretched arms.
3. Perform back stretches and strengthening exercises daily, recognizing that strong abdominals is the key to preventing back pain.
4. Maintain ideal body weight.
5. Can sleeping cause back pain?

We spend about one third of our time in bed. Therefore, we cannot ignore how our bodies are positioned during sleep. We need to maintain a neutral spine even while we are in bed.

HERE ARE MY TIPS FOR SLEEPING:

1. Make sure you are sleeping on a comfortable mattress. I don't recommend a water bed. It does not provide enough support. Try out the mattress before you buy it. Just because it costs a lot, doesn't mean it is the right one for you.

2. Avoid sleeping on your stomach or with your head elevated on an oversized pillow. These positions cause the back to arch and places stress on the spine.

3. Sleeping on the side and back are the best positions for maintaining a neutral position.

4. Place a pillow between your knees (for side sleeping) or behind your knees (for back sleeping). This will help keep your spine in the right position and help ease the stress on the lower back.

5. Use a pillow that allows you to keep your head aligned with the rest of your body.

6. Avoid oversized pillows. They may be decorative, but they do not benefit your back while sleeping.

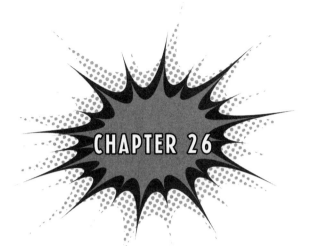

Common Exercises to Relieve Back Pain

Keep Your Back Flexible and Strong:
Do these Exercises Three to Five Times per Week

1. PELVIC TILT

Flatten back by tightening stomach muscles and buttocks. Repeat 30 times per set. Do one set each day.

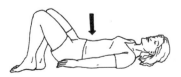

2. LOWER TRUNK
ROTATION STRETCH

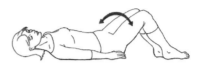

Keeping back flat and feet

together, rotate knees to right/left side. Hold for 20 to 30

seconds and repeat five times per set. Do one set each day.

3. KNEE TO CHEST
STRETCH (UNILATERAL)

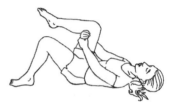

With the hand behind the knee,

pull the knee toward the chest until you feel a comfortable

stretch in the lower back and buttocks. Try to keep back re-

laxed. Hold 20 to 30 seconds and repeat five times. Do these

once a day (especially good for stenosis).

4. BRIDGING

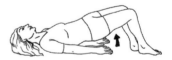

Slowly raise buttocks from floor, keeping stomach tight. Re-

peat 30 times. Do these once a day.

5. PARTIAL SIT-UP

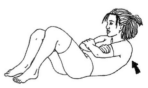

Keeping arms folded across chest,

tilt pelvis to flatten back. Raise

head and shoulders from the floor. Repeat 10 times. Do three sets per session, one session each day.

Remember: strong abdominals are the KEY to a healthy back. Ask your doctor if this one is okay for you.

6. UPPER/LOWER EXTREMITY EXTENSION

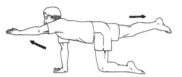

While on all fours, tighten the stomach and raise right/left leg and opposite arm. Keep back rigid. Repeat 10 times per set. Do two sets per session, do one session per day. Repeat three to four times per week.

7. HAMSTRING STRETCH

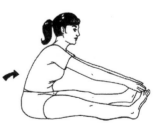

While sitting on the floor, reach forward and touch the toes of each leg until a comfortable stretch is felt in back of the thigh. Do not bend the knee. Hold for 30 seconds, repeat five times per set. Do one set each day. If this is difficult, extend one leg at at time to stretch one hamstring. Hold 20 to 30 seconds.

8. QUADRICEPS STRETCH

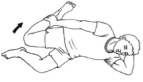

While lying on the floor, roll on your side, pull right/left heel in toward the buttocks until a comfortable stretch is felt in front of the thigh. Hold 20 to 30 seconds, repeat five times. Do these stretches once a day.

9. HAMSTRING STRETCH

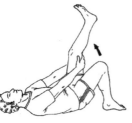

While lying supine on the floor, put your hand behind the right/left knee. Start with the knee bent, and attempt to straighten the knee until a comfortable stretch is felt in back of the thigh. Hold 20 to 30 seconds, repeat five times. Do once each day.

10. BACKWARD BEND

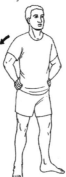

While standing, place hands on the hips and arch the back backward. Hold for 5 seconds. Repeat 10 times. Can be done multiple times during the day.

If an exercise increases your back pain after five repetitions, stop. Consult your doctor before starting any exercise program.

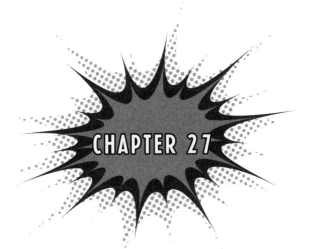

CHAPTER 27

Resource Sheets

Keep track of your health.

 onitor your body weight and exercise program with these charts to monitor your progress. These tables will help you to visualize your progress.

WEEKLY BODY WEIGHT

Dates						

WEEKLY EXERCISES/ACTIVITIES

Exercise	M	T	W	T	F	S	S
Walking	2 miles						
Gardening		2 hours		1 hour			

RESOURCES

Some of the products I have recommended over the years:

- Aspen semirigid back braces
- McKenzie lumbar rolls
- Gel ice packs

To learn more about various orthopedic conditions, please visit our website at **www.knockoutpain.com**. and sign up for our monthly tips.

Feel free to contact us at **info@knockoutpain.com.**

Visit our Youtube channel for Dr. Winifred Bragg to see what others are saying about our comprehensive approach to treating their back pain.

CONTACT DR. BRAGG

Dr. Bragg frequently speaks on strategies to help you Turn Pain to Power™ using the Bragg Factor® a system that provides a blueprint to help you reach your maximum potential in your personal or professional life. She can deliver a keynote speech customized to meet your needs. She has been the keynote speaker at programs such as the "Take Your Daughters to Work" national program, which was held at the US Capitol.

If you are interested in finding out more, please visit her speaking page at **www.DrBraggSpeaks.com** or her practice website at **www.knockoutpain.com**.

This book is available for quantity discounts for bulk purchases. Please contact us at www.knockoutpain.com

ABOUT WINIFRED BRAGG, MD

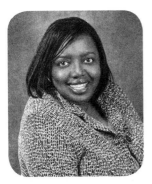 Dr. Bragg is an expert in providing nonsurgical treatment for injuries and pain resulting from spinal and orthopedic conditions. She has treated thousands of patients successfully by providing a comprehensive approach to their pain by using customized treatment plans. A nationally recognized speaker, Dr. Bragg has appeared in numerous TV and print media programs and has been featured on ABC, NBC, CBS and FOX. She has been quoted as an expert in *Redbook* ("The New Way to Beat Back Pain"); *Women's World* ("Get Rid of Backache for Good"); *Weight Watcher's Magazine* ("Back on Track"); *Newark Sunday Star-Ledger* ("To Your Health: Oh, Her Aching Back"); and *Self Magazine* ("A Pain in the Back"). She is board certified both in Physical Medicine and Rehabilitation and Pain Medicine.

Dr. Bragg received her undergraduate degree from the University of Alabama, her medical degree from Meharry Medical College, and completed an internship at the Baptist Medical Center in Birmingham. She completed her residency training at the University of Michigan. Additionally, she completed an internship in the Office of the United States Surgeon General. She is the Medical Director of the Spine and Orthopedic Pain Center and has offices in Norfolk and Chesapeake, Virginia.

For more information, please visit our website at
www.knockoutpain.com